Advance Pr

"I am so impressed with how Julie was able to use her own devastating experience to develop a practical but nurturing perspective that she can share with others struggling with fertility issues. Her book transcends "how to get pregnant" advice, and instead guides women in an exploration of ways that they can work through the debilitating sadness that often comes when women are desperately trying to get pregnant. Her book is filled with grace and compassion for women facing some of the most frustrating, heartbreaking challenges."

- Toni Weschler, MPH
Author of *Taking Charge of Your Fertility*

"Honest, compassionate, readable and transformative…the author courageously shares her journey through infertility to her own rebirth. Both women and men would greatly benefit from reading this powerful expose of real issues around fertility and parenthood. Wise guidance for aligning heart, mind and body in the journey to parenthood."

- Dr. Susan M. Engman, Psychologist

"There is currently so much noise about infertility and what is not possible, and we often lose how personal each story is. In *I Still Want to be a Mom*, Julie Pierce offers a fresh and unique perspective that may help with the questions, struggles, and emotions women have when fertility becomes a challenge."

- Samuel Tong, M.Sc., D.C.

"Reading this book provides great clarity into the journey of infertility. Julie's insight is incredibly honest, thoughtful, and reaches the reader on a personal level. This book reminded me of my own experience working with Julie, which helped me find a road back to hope, acceptance, and joy."

- Laura Colic, happy mom and client

"Julie Pierce's *I still want to Be a Mom* is the book to read as you navigate your way on the road of fertility. Julie's own challenges through this process makes her an excellent guide because she's been there! She will lovingly connect you back to your heart's desire while empowering you to focus on you as a whole person because it's more than just eggs, uterus, and sperm. Let her guidance light the way for you."

- Jackie Foskett, Hypnotherapist, Stress Relief Specialist Author of *The Stress Relief Toolbox: For Women Who Take Care of Everyone But Themselves*

"Julie Pierce gives practical tools to start changing your relationship with your body and self when the journey to becoming a mom is rougher than expected. *I Still Want to Be a Mom* will lead you back to the unconditional love out of which new life grows."

- Sharon Pope, The Love & Relationship Coach for Women Who Want More, SharonPopeTruth.com Master Life Coach and Six-Time International Best-Selling Author

"We are encouraged to see a book like *I Still Want To Be A Mom* include a full acknowledgment of the role grief can often play in reproduction. That Julie has incorporated creative grief techniques for people to realize a full range of emotion and process on this path is a gift for families seeking this type of support."

- Cath Duncan & Kara Jones, CreativeGriefStudio.com

I Still Want to be a Mom

I Still Want to be a 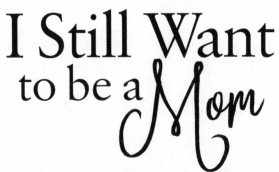Mom

Escaping Hopelessness
& Embracing Motherhood

Julie A. Pierce

NEW YORK

LONDON • NASHVILLE • MELBOURNE • VANCOUVER

I Still Want to be a Mom

Escaping Hopelessness and Embracing Motherhood

Published in New York, New York, by Morgan James Publishing in partnership with Difference Press. Morgan James is a trademark of Morgan James, LLC. www.MorganJamesPublishing.com

The Morgan James Speakers Group can bring authors to your live event. For more information or to book an event visit The Morgan James Speakers Group at www.TheMorganJamesSpeakersGroup.com.

ISBN 9781683506959 paperback
ISBN 9781683506966 eBook
Library of Congress Control Number: 2017911887

Cover Design by:
Rachel Lopez
www.r2cdesign.com

Interior Design by:
Chris Treccani
www.3dogcreative.net

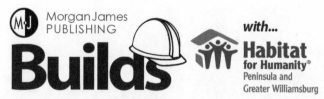

In an effort to support local communities, raise awareness and funds, Morgan James Publishing donates a percentage of all book sales for the life of each book to Habitat for Humanity Peninsula and Greater Williamsburg.

Get involved today! Visit
www.MorganJamesBuilds.com

For Christopher and Ava, who profoundly blessed my life.

Table of Contents

Introduction

Another Book About Infertility? No, Not Really

You've picked up another book with the hope that it might get you closer to parenthood. But it's looking pretty glum. I know it's painful. Not so long ago, I was right there where you are, in that pain and uncertainty, feeling overwhelmed and in despair. I'm not there anymore, but I assure you, I remember it well.

From Excited Desire to Overwhelmed Despair

Like the one person who shows up at the party on the wrong day, you feel like a lonely fool, and you're no longer sure you'll bother to go to the party after all. I promise you that you are not alone and you are not a fool. Lots of women like you and me go through this every day, but it's kept under wraps. We're all busy living lives that look like they should be Pinterest boards – but we all know that's not real.

Let's get real. Let's talk about what *really* happens. I'll start the conversation with some of my story, and let's see if it's similar to yours.

Once upon a time, I was a girl growing up in a world that told me the only limits I had were the ones I put on myself. I had ambitions; I was going places and making things happen. I felt that I had big things to do even if I wasn't sure what those things were. I just knew I was going to make an impact and life was good.

I understood that it was my responsibility to make it to adulthood and create a life supported by my own efforts before even considering becoming a mom. I noticed that there were threats to my ambitions already surrounding me – cultural norms, intimate relationships, and opportunities for "too much fun." I stayed focused. I went to college; I got a job; I made my way into adulthood on what looked like a great trajectory.

Even though I always felt a natural affection for children – and had an unspoken understanding that I'd be a mom someday – I was very active and vigilant about not allowing myself to get pregnant. No way was this going to happen to me. The timing and the situation would need to be right before I could entertain the possibility of motherhood. And the values that I inherited told me I had to be married and financially stable so I could support my children.

I got married at 27. And as soon as I had mailed the last thank you note for wedding gifts, I was getting enquiries about my schedule for making Junior. What?!

By the time I was 30, the question got louder. I was also feeling the gravity of the popular focus on how aging impacts fertility and pregnancy. I experienced massive conflict and confusion. Family added their own salty expectations, with comments that women who choose not to be moms are selfish. Yikes! I didn't want to be that. Yet, I wasn't sure I was ready to commit to the responsibilities of motherhood. I entered the spin cycle of confusion, obligation, fear, and overwhelm … and this was before the repeatedly failed attempts at conception, and then the miscarriage, and finally stillbirth.

Misery and struggle … grief and isolation. There was definitely something wrong with me, but being the girl who always had her life together, there was no way I'd let anyone know what a hot mess I really was. I was even keeping my husband at arm's length about my inner turmoil. And then when we brought in the experts in assisted reproductive technology, the distance between me and Scott grew even larger. I felt so alone … which made no sense because reproduction takes two, right?

I was in despair big time. There was a mountain of decisions and I was trying to make them alone. Although I didn't realize it, I really needed someone to help me deal with the ups and downs – the building up of hope *again* and the defeat and grief of the negative pregnancy test *again*. I was angry and frustrated by the responses that the doctors were giving me. Their "answers" weren't satisfying and they didn't always make sense. They were not moving me forward.

I was concerned that I was using medications that weren't really helping me get pregnant and that might be, even worse, causing more reproductive trouble. I had a sense that there was a bigger problem at hand that I needed to address in order for me to get pregnant and bring home my healthy baby.

I didn't know what the problem was, but if I could figure it out, then I would know what I needed to do. I just wanted to confidently understand what my realistic options were, and I felt like no one was giving me an answer I could put money on.

Was I wasting time trying to conceive? Was this even an option for me? Or was I making my conception even more difficult with the medications and treatments that I was just going along with? I felt like I was running out of time, and the right information was still eluding me. I was overwhelmed, confused, frustrated, and exhausted.

I didn't want to let my husband down. He said that whether it happened or not, he'd be happy either way, lovingly reassuring me that he appreciated our relationship no matter what. He tried to take the pressure off me. But it was hard for him to understand all the pieces. He was as supportive as he could be; he was frustrated too.

A lot of my friends were already happily busy with the occupation of motherhood and couldn't relate, and the friends that weren't moms didn't really understand either. I wanted to be able to share what I was going through with them, but I felt embarrassed. I didn't really want their advice; I just wanted them to listen and hear what I was going through – without them thinking I was pathetic.

Once I realized that conceiving was going to be more difficult than I imagined, I got very concerned with things I hadn't thought of before. Like biological time constraints – I felt like the months were loudly ticking away. I felt disappointment with myself. My body was not working the way it should. I felt betrayed. Other friends and family members became pregnant easily.

I felt I was failing my husband; I knew that he really wanted to be a dad. And I was failing myself. I wanted to scream, "Why can't my body just work the way it's supposed to?" I was on the edge of self-loathing, and that seemed so pathetically dramatic, but it was also true. The meds made me feel physically and emotionally crazy.

I was not ready to accept that motherhood wasn't going to happen for me. I rejected the word "infertility" – it was a death knell to hope. I was constantly searching for and gathering shards and shadows of possibility. I was not ready to let it go. I thought I should just try harder, putting more demands on myself to improve.

Can you relate to any of this? If you do, I'm sorry you're going through this, and I want you to know it doesn't have to be this way.

When I lost my daughter in my third trimester, I asked myself, "What's the point?" I literally wanted to die. And then, it all turned. I had a huge shift.

Things got easier, better, lighter. I want that for you before you reach the point of "give up or die."

What Makes This Book Different?

In this book, I'm not going to give you gloomy statistics and reality checks about your age and the quality of your eggs. I'm not going to tell you to forget the pursuit of having your own child and go directly to considering adoption. I'm also not going to tell you that you need assisted reproductive technology. Any of these might work for you, but I'm not going to pretend to know what your best answer is.

What makes this book different and valuable is that it opens an opportunity for you to gain an effective alternative perspective on how you are approaching your dream of motherhood. It offers unique insight into an under-the-skin, deep-down view at an energetic level of what's going on with your fertility.

This is how I work with my clients. This is how so many women have come to me, feeling broken and in despair. We work together and lights come on. The path forward becomes more clear. Hope is renewed. Energy is regained. Babies are born. I want that for you too.

Should You Dare to Hope?

In one word, yes! I believe you have the courage for this challenge. You're already here. You wouldn't be picking up this book if you didn't have the required courage. If you're still thinking now is the time for you to be a mom, I want you to know this challenge will not kill you no matter how difficult it feels. I can say that confidently from personal experience and from witnessing the triumphs of my clients who, yes, *dare* to hope.

My Promise to You

Your heart gives you a desire not to torture you, but to lead you in the direction of fulfilling the promises of your life. Your soul is speaking to you. This is no longer an intellectual exercise. It's much deeper than that. And it does require courage. Things can naturally clear when we trust in and follow the messages of the heart and body.

If you will engage the infinite possibility that is yours and stay connected with your desire and your courage, things can be different for you too. I promise that if you open yourself to what I'm offering you, things will begin to change. Something will shift, and you will no longer be experiencing the struggle you are in right now.

Part 1

MY STORY AND
THREE BIG MISTAKES

"It's snowing still," said Eeyore gloomily.
"So it is."
"And freezing."
"Is it?"
"Yes," said Eeyore. "However," he said, brightening up a little,
"we haven't had an earthquake lately."

- excerpt from *The House At Pooh Corner*,
by A.A. Milne

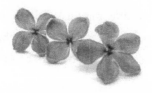

Chapter 1
An Initiation by Fire into Peace

Everything Comes Easy Until It Doesn't

Has anyone ever told you that everything comes easily to you? I heard those words, and I took them in like a curse. I could see how the person who said this to me might think that, but I'd had my fair share of difficulties, and I'd grown some deep-rooted resilience as a result. I am grateful for that. Resilience is a superpower.

Although my childhood had some tumultuous episodes between my parents' divorces and my growing up overseas between the ages of 9 and 18, my life did appear to be pretty smooth and full of sweetness. The acrid flavors are in the details, and that's not really what I chose to highlight when I told my story.

I was a college graduate with an appreciation for exotic and global encounters. I was embarking on the next phase of life alongside the man who would years later become my husband. There was a lot of laughter and ambition in my belly, and I had a sense that I could literally do anything. I got my first corporate job about a year after graduation, and then my career really took off.

We were the typical aspiring yuppies and our budget was finally beginning to catch up with our lifestyle. Eventually we got married, proudly paying for our own homegrown, modest wedding. And then we invested in our first property – a tiny condo. We felt we were on the path to success, and we were lovin' life.

Soon after the last wedding gift thank you note was mailed, people started asking, "So when do you think you'll have a kid?" Friends, family, people I just met – it felt like this question was on everyone's minds except ours.

I was not ready to consider the issue. I did not have a burning desire to be a mom yet, and my husband just wanted to do whatever would make me happy. Despite our lack of clarity around parenting, we were aligned in our values, believing that before embarking on parenthood we should be financially stable, responsible adults. Whatever that meant.

You Just Decide and Then Have Sex, Right?

So, there we were – the happy couple. Time went by, as time does. And then, three years into marriage and eight years into our relationship, we began to give a sideways glance to the question of parenthood. We had the house and the jobs, but did we have the desire? Each of us was still noncommittal. Besides, I was getting ready to change careers. Was this really a good time? And what was happening with the economy?

We tossed those questions to the wind and decided to give it shot. We'd swing the door wide open to the possibility by eliminating prevention. How very daring of us!

It seemed so vulnerable, and surprisingly scary – we were literally unprotected. Perhaps our natures naturally leaned too far to the side of sober responsibility. We had to work at being comfortable with the possibility of conception. I'm sure this is not how it's supposed to be, right? As you might have guessed, it wasn't happening.

Really, Really Ready?

In retrospect, I can see that we really did not feel ready. All my fears about being a good parent and not wanting to raise my child alone – as if there was even a threat that my husband would leave – were living large in my head. Crazy notions that had brewed strong and deep inside me, created a thick residue of a different kind of protection. Clearly I was not really, really ready.

Looking for the Universe's "Yes"

On trend with what felt like our very uncharacteristic turn toward complete irresponsibility, my husband and I agreed that if it happened that would be super cool, but we weren't going to get attached to making it happen. We'd let the Universe decide. What we forgot is that the Universe simply reacts and provides what's in alignment with your heart. So if your heart is not clear, there is no delivery.

We looked for a Yes from the Universe for a good long time; and we thought it was delivering a No. We were wrong. We were delivering the No. We tortured ourselves with conflicting messages. On the one hand, we were intensely vigilant about my cycles, and on the other hand we were completely nonchalant about what we wanted. The conflicted message was, "We're totally committed, but we don't really care."

Fence Sitting

This was fence sitting at its finest and most inconspicuous. It didn't *appear* that we were on the fence. We were only talking about it between ourselves, but we never had a real, direct discussion with the clear conclusion of a Yes or a No to the question, "Do you want to have a baby?"

Even when I pretended that I had made a decision, I wasn't sure about Scott's desires, and so I second-guessed my own. I didn't want to lose the beautiful relationship we had created between just the two of us. I liked that we had cats as kiddos. Although cats have attitudes, we could easily meet their needs and feel good about our parenting.

Because I was approaching my mid-30s, we felt the weight of the popular stance that we had to do it now if we were going to do it at all. And so we began in earnest with the clear goal of pregnancy. We committed to trying our best, swinging for the fences. But we were still seeing disappointing results on the home pregnancy tests.

My doctor told me she thought maybe I had endometriosis after finding nothing else to hang our hat on. I felt very clear that I did not. And sure enough, after investigation, I turned out to be correct.

The fertility drugs I had tried were not the answer for me either. They made me feel crazy, and I had not conceived. The next step in the progression through the medical establishment led to the auspices of assisted reproductive technology. And that was a road I was not ready to travel – yet.

So I went back to denying the grief that accompanied my monthly menstruation. I resumed trying to convince myself that I didn't really care, and that being childless was really what I wanted.

We did talk adoption for about two seconds, and we decided to reserve the fullness of that conversation for "later," more desperate, times. We didn't feel we had arrived at those times just yet. I'm not sure what we were waiting for.

Every now and then there seemed to be a ray of hope forming when my period was late. But the crash that came with the arrival of red was a loud emotional pain.

There was a very early miscarriage. And then there was an early but more significant miscarriage. I had always considered myself the expert of my body, and I was less interested in the opinions of doctors since the "you might have endometriosis" encounter. But through the progression of these experiences of loss, my belief that I was able to conceive was growing. After all, I had to conceive before I could miscarry. It felt like I was warming up or finally making it to the starting line. At the same time, my fear of what conceiving would really mean was also growing.

Handing Over Faith

Then the picture of what was happening to me emotionally on a regular monthly basis clicked into 3D, Technicolor focus. I was riding up and down on a roller coaster every month, and the down part began with the arrival of my period. The grief of another month when conception didn't happen would hit me hard.

As my period ended, my tears would dry and I'd become emotionally resigned to reality. Then I'd move from resigned ambivalence to sheer relief, wondering how and why I had gotten so torn up about it in the first place. I would enjoy conversations with girlfriends who were clear that they didn't want to be moms, engaging with our visions of how free our lives would always be without kids in tow.

And then a few days before ovulation, I would be struck by a spell that had me searching for puppies and kittens and babies to cuddle. It was an irrational longing that felt like it came from the deepest place within my soul. It made me feel like a crazy person. My obsession with conceiving was powerfully renewed. I had to be a mother! It was a soul imperative.

And then my period would once again herald the news that in fact there would be no baby, and I would be devastated. And then back to the place of ambivalence and relief. And then obsession to devastation, and so on. I felt unsettlingly unstable.

At my next gyno check-up, I decided to ask about this crazy pattern with the doc. I trusted this doctor; she was different. She offered just the right mix of wielding medical authority and respecting *my* authority over knowing my body. She gave me the biggest gift a doctor had ever given me up to that point in my life.

She looked me in the eye and told me I was indeed not crazy. Rather, I was perfectly in tune with my hormonal cycle and, given the intensity of my emotional response to the ovulation stage, she felt it was safe to say that I had a very large space in my heart for a child. She quickly followed that up by supporting me in understanding my options and following the path that felt most right for me.

We concluded that since I was now 36, I should go to a fertility clinic, run some additional labs, and form a plan based on their recommendations. She referred me to a specific colleague. That's who I called. That's who I saw. That's who I put my faith in going forward. It was a turning point for me. There was a sense of excited anticipation that I hadn't felt for a while, but it was mixed with apprehension and revulsion. I wanted to vomit.

Because of these mixed feelings and my confusing, conflicted desire around being a mother, I decided to see the counselor at the fertility clinic. What I was looking for was a way to feel confidently clear about my desire to be a mom. I felt that if I could nail that down, the rest would naturally unfold. I would clearly recognize the right next step from an internal source of wisdom, not from an external source of lab results. Unfortunately, the counseling aggravated my feelings of overwhelm rather than bringing any resolution.

And so there I was, deeper in confusion, except for the monthly beacon of clear direction that I received during ovulation. I decided to follow that beacon. I thought that it was time to give in to the final frontier that I had been strongly resisting for so long.

And that's how I moved away from faith in myself and my body and handed it all over to the gods of medical science to make my body bring me a baby. It began with more tests. Results showed that there was no conclusive evidence for why I was not getting pregnant. Awesome! Still no real answer. However, the reproductive authorities informed my husband and me that IUI (intrauterine insemination) could be just the ticket to get the sperm and the egg to collaborate in ways they currently weren't. That only half made sense to me given the miscarriages. But I reminded myself that I was handing it all over to them now, so I went along with it through three cycles. Nothing.

The next step recommended by the fertility doc was IVF (in vitro fertilization). My reaction to the suggestion was a full-body freeze. I really wasn't ready to accept this next step just yet.

All my feelings of failure returned. My hope had grown strong over the course of the three IUI cycles. Yet ultimately it was crushed again. Meanwhile, my husband was standing by waiting for my decision of what to do next. I felt so alone in the decision-making, and the idea that there was a right and a wrong answer was powerfully paralyzing. I wasn't sure what to make of it all. I had so many questions without any satisfactory answers. I just wanted to run away from everyone, including myself.

After a couple of months went by, I began to buy into the belief that this was my very last chance. The clincher came when a friend told me casually at lunch one day, "Your eggs aren't getting any younger." From her perspective, she couldn't understand why I hadn't gone directly to IVF without hesitation. How could she understand? She had two beautiful girls, both conceived naturally without a sneeze of difficulty. And I loved and trusted this friend. So I was ready to believe that she was right.

I also rationalized that if I tried IVF and it failed, then I was getting that clear No from the Universe that I had been looking for so many years ago. I could feel resolved that I had tried everything I could, and there would be nothing else to do to my body to coax it into what its parts were naturally made to do.

And Now We Make a Baby – Initial Surrender

The make-a-baby lab kit arrived on my doorstep from the pharmaceutical distributor associated with the fertility clinic. It contained an assortment of needles and syringes, injectable pens, pills, liquid solutions, sterile cleansing wipes, and the itemized invoice. Once again, I experienced the full-body freeze. The words that came to mind were, "Frankenstein baby."

I was having reservations. I decided that I would feel better, stronger, if I took control of the scary box's contents – let those contents know who was in charge here. I took everything out of the box and grabbed a sharpie and the IVF calendar from the clinic. I marked each box and bottle with schedule information and put the items that needed refrigeration into the fridge. I organized the other items in my bathroom and prepared myself to make the presentation to Scott when he got home from work.

With my husband's help, I got into a groove with the schedule of pills and shots. And then something weird and unexpected happened. A calm sense of control and certainty came over me like I hadn't experienced for a long time. I had a knowing that I was going to get pregnant this time and it was going to be game on. I gave in to the process – initial surrender. It felt good to be doing something that I knew would be effective. I just knew. This was very different feeling for me. During all the other attempts, I never felt certainty like this.

And so it came to be that I was pregnant. The message from the clinic following the two weeks after the IVF procedure told us that we were to be cautiously optimistic. That the growth factor measurement was on the right trajectory, but it was early days, of course.

And then at eight weeks we got to see the most amazing thing in the whole world – our baby's heartbeat. My mind was literally blown. There she was, my baby. Growing. From an embryo, to a fetus, to a baby. With arms and legs and a face.

I looked at her so many times between weeks eight and twenty-seven. Sometimes as a flat gray and white image and sometimes as a golden-orange moving 3D image. In my eyes, she was always beautiful, even when she looked like E.T.

During the middle of my pregnancy with Ava, I would have moments of being curiously overcome with great grief that felt like the grief of millennia of women who had come before me. And at the same time as I was visited by this great grief, I had a sense of being surrounded by female ancestors from all time, holding us grieving ones in comfort, witnessing and catching our tears. It was peculiar to me – what was I grieving about? There was nothing I could do but give in to those moments and the flood of tears. I consoled myself that it was just part of my process. I breathed through it, let the tears and feelings flow, and focused on my gratitude for the time I was savoring as new life grew inside me.

The Unimagined

Finally, my third trimester dawned. I celebrated that the finish line was in sight; I would hold my baby in my arms soon and gaze into her eyes.

It was three weeks exactly since I had last seen my beautiful baby girl via ultrasound, moving like the tiny dancer that she was. That day I met a friend for lunch. I parked, got out of my car, and began to walk toward the restaurant. And then there was an earthquake inside of me.

In that instant, I understood that I had lost her. But I would not accept this information. I went on to my lunch meeting. I ate and talked and laughed and pretended that all was well … but I knew.

I smiled when I saw my husband come home that night. We went out for dinner with friends. Again, I ate and talked and laughed and pretended all was well … but I knew.

When we got home from dinner, I told my husband about my earthquake. I also told him that I was hopeful all was well, and I would give her until morning to move before I called the hospital. But I knew.

At 4:00 am I had had enough knowing and no doing. I got out of bed. Took the fastest shower in the history of time and called the hospital. They told me to come in for a non-stress test, more accurately referred to as fetal heart rate monitoring. But I already knew.

My husband was starting a new job that morning with an important meeting. I told him I'd be fine to go alone, and I'd call him if I needed him.

My senses were keen and everything was in brighter color than usual. It felt like I could smell and hear everything near and far.

I walked onto the labor and delivery floor and saw a sea of blue uniforms. I walked up to the desk and with a forced smile said, "Hi. I'm Julie Pierce. I called. I'm here for a non-stress test, and I'm trying not to be stressed." No one laughed at my sad joke. I was quickly ushered into a room and a monitor was wheeled in. The nurse had me lay on the bed. The monitor screen was facing away from me. But I already knew.

The nurse's face showed concern while she ran the wand through the jelly slathered over my exposed belly. And then without making eye contact, she put the wand down and said, "I'll be right back with the doctor."

It was fine. I already knew.

The doctor came in with an austere air about her. She looked at the monitor while running the wand through the jelly. And then, without looking at me, she said, "I'm sorry, but there's no heartbeat."

And to my surprise, although I already knew, I screamed at her, "That can't be!"

She swung the monitor screen to face me and tersely said, "Well, it's true. Look at it for yourself." And then she left the room. I was devastated – I felt miserably and sharply broken and alone.

Mercifully, an angel in the form of a nurse named Rose came into my room, sat down on the bed beside me, and held me while the tears poured out of my eyes and my body shook with sobs. Another nurse came into the room to ask if I wanted to call my husband. I couldn't speak. The nurse offered to call him for me. I handed her my phone.

And so my bad-news truth began to spread. It was in that moment of the message leaving that room that I truly understood how speaking something makes it more real. This was the deepest pain I have ever felt.

Full, Active Surrender

According to Traditional Chinese Medicine (TCM), after the loss of a baby during pregnancy, the body and spirit require a length of time equal to the length of time that the pregnancy was held before it's recommended to conceive again. My acupuncturist said this to me and I heard her, but I wasn't ready to think about or feel into the possibility of another pregnancy when she told me. And then I forgot about the time frame. I forgot about a lot of logical things. I went to a deep and dark place once I realized that people were getting tired of me sharing the story of my pregnancy loss and the birth of my daughter Ava Catherine.

Even my husband wanted to stop talking about her. The world was moving on as it does; I wasn't ready. I took my time to re-member myself. I did a lot of moaning and crying into a pillow, deep-soul sobs that I had never experienced before. I also did a lot of sleeping. And when social interaction was necessary, I did a lot of acting.

Time passed. My body healed. The shattered pieces of my heart grew back together.

Finally, the question of whether I would try again came into my awareness. Yes, I really should look at this question if I was ever going to have a baby of my own. I was 39 years old now and as one of my dear friends said, "Tick tock." I spent many weeks going inward, asking this question of my heart and soul, waiting and listening for an answer.

And then, I noticed how peaceful and quiet things had gotten for me. I noticed that I felt stronger in a way that I had not known before – more solid and clear. I had lived through my own natural disaster. I had survived the most devastating experience of my life – a nightmare I had never imagined. I was still here.

I felt the desire for motherhood beating loudly in my heart. Yes, I would do this again.

The best way I can describe the overarching feeling of this transition from broken down to rising again is *surrender*. I gave myself up to whatever would be. This new experience of peace and certainty came from a knowing that I still had and continue to have value to offer the world no matter what the outcome of this pursuit would ultimately be.

I knew what I had to do; I knew how to do it; and I knew what the range of possible outcomes could be. I showed up with a "Yes, let's do this," in calm, peaceful surrender of myself to the faith that I am perfect and whole no matter the circumstances I encounter. I am here, present in this lifetime; I want to live and contribute. I recognized that I can do what I know how to do and that the rest is completely out of my control.

I hadn't ever had the felt-sense clarity like this before. With this new and profound understanding, I was ready and prepared to get pregnant and carry myself and my baby into motherhood like I had never been ready before. And when I checked the calendar, I was right on time regarding the recommendations of TCM.

It's a faith walk in a wide, infinite field of possible outcomes. I would walk the path that was uniquely mine knowing that I would arrive at my perfect destination – and what that was would be unknown to me till I got there. I was comfortable with the uncertain parts from that moment forward. What I *was* certain about was that I would move forward and this process would not be the end of me. The fear and conflict were gone.

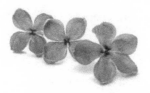

Chapter 2

Three Common Mistakes: Fast Track to Fragile Fertility

B y reflecting on my own journey and by observing the women I work with, I notice a trend of three common mistakes that perpetuate our struggle and lead to defeat. I see this happen even when we think we're doing the right things to get our bodies to deliver us a baby. What you may find surprising is that there is much more to this puzzle than eggs, sperm, hormones, and a uterus.

These words may feel a bit harsh as you read them, but I write them to you with the intention to lovingly reveal something new to you. I know this from the inside out. I've been there. You may reject what I write to you here, or you may find a dawning of a new kind of understanding. My wish is that you receive an opening up rather than a shutting down from what I share here. You may be able to identify these three mistakes and growth points reflected in the story of my journey that I shared in the previous chapter.

Pride of Control

I've encountered many women like me struggling with fertility challenges and working at baby-making like it's a project we manage at work. The idea is that it should fit into a life schedule. However, making and growing a baby is a movement of collaborative creation and ultimately a surrender into faith. It's like being part of a choir.

Being the lead singer and controlling the direction of the song doesn't work; rather, it throws the song into disarray. Your job is to sing the words in the agreed-upon rhythm in the agreed-upon key and, in faith that by doing just the part that is yours to do, collaboratively create a beautiful song. You can only sing your part. You cannot create the beautiful sound without a collaborative relationship with the choir.

The mistake is in believing you can control all the elements and therefore the outcome. Control likes to ride on cold strategy. Strategy is head-driven. Baby-making comes from a harmony of heart, soul, body, and mind. Strategy may guide actions, but it alone does not make a baby.

Punishment of Body and Spirit

Another common defeating practice that I engaged in and that I've witnessed over and over again is how we punish our bodies – and consequently our spirits. This often happens once we've taken on the task of baby-making like we are on a crusade. It's a consequence of the first mistake, Pride of Control.

We are brutal to the very being we need as our most vital ally: our body. All the poking and prodding with exams and lab tests and the performance-on-demand requirements … all this physical intrusion and coercion sets up a dynamic of contraction and shrinking. The body refuses to perform; it rebels. A hardness sets in. A baby cannot grow on a hard surface. This scenario is the opposite of warm, nurturing, soft reception.

We make unrelenting demands on our soil without giving the love, sunlight, and water it needs to produce the beautiful fruit we are dreaming about. This is as crazy as riding a horse through the desert without giving it any water, and then kicking it when it falls down, yelling, "Get up, worthless horse! We're not there yet!"

Prejudice for the Conflict

There's a third self-generated mechanism that is the hardest to see, accept, and change in ourselves. This is the tricky, slippery one where the subconscious mind expertly does its job of maintaining our thought habits and patterns, protecting us from the truth of ourselves. You see, if we could discern the truth of our thought habits and patterns, we would more confidently make choices about whether we really want to make the changes that need to happen so that we can be the person who does become a mother in the way we are imagining.

This might sound a bit esoteric, so let's bring it down to earth. What we are talking about here is first grappling with the need for certainty, and then becoming experts at how we can actually create our own certainty.

Ultimately, the only certainty that we can experience is what we generate from the inside – with our minds and hearts. This certainty comes from what we believe. There is value in being able to answer the question, "Am I deceiving myself with beliefs that conflict with my desires? Are my beliefs giving me certainty about what I fear or about what I want?" Whatever you believe – whether it supports you or undermines you – will always be true for you.

Beliefs are the foundation for our capacity to commit to the pursuit of a desire, all the while accepting that the outcome is uncertain and out of our direct control. The outcome is uncertain because it is outside of us. But we often fall into the trap of not accepting this kind of uncertainty. This non-acceptance perpetuates our prejudice for our own conflicting beliefs and desires, and this conflict keeps us stuck and struggling.

We run on the hamster wheel of repetitive thought habits and patterns that lead us to repeat what is not working for us. This leads to more frustration and paralysis when faced with new choices and decisions. We become so overwhelmed that we check out, disconnecting from ourselves, from our body, and from those who love us. And there we are, discouraged and isolated, experiencing our beautiful desire as a torturous longing.

It truly doesn't have to be this way.

Now it's your turn. Look into your experience and see if you can recognize any of these three patterns that I've described here. Beware. The third one can make it almost impossible to see the other two.

Part 2

MENDING WHAT'S BROKEN

*"Every change in the human physiological state is accompanied by
an appropriate change in the mental-emotional state, conscious or
unconscious, and conversely every change in the human mental-emotional
state, conscious or unconscious, is accompanied by an appropriate change
in the physiological state."*

– The Psychophysiological Principle,
Elmer and Alyce Green

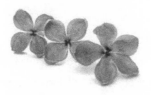

Chapter 3
Myths and Miracles of Biochemistry

Most of us know someone who got preggo in high school, despite the warnings of a doomed life and the strained communications about prevention. That fact seems to have proven how easy it is to do this thing; how inevitable it is that having sex results in a baby.

But now that we're in the struggle of pursuing motherhood, it looks like we were sold a lie. This lie and other influences induced fear, and fear has established inter-fear-ence in the body-mind cooperative mechanism. There's some untangling and sorting to do here before we can proceed. So take a deep breath while we unmuddle and find a baseline understanding of the facts. From there, we can confidently consider next steps.

Required Elements

First let's get clear on the minimal physical requirements for the baby-making project. Let's also understand what we can influence to improve our odds of bringing home a healthy baby. And if you're thinking, "But I've already read this in every fertility book I've already read," that's cool. I'm going to bottom-line each of these so you know if any of them are a concern for you. If you're already perfectly clear on this part, skim it or skip ahead to the section Beyond the Body. I also recommend reading and really understanding the sections Stress Hormones and Good Eggs.

In the brief quiz, How Fertile Are You?, I walk you through some questions to gauge where you are on the fertility spectrum from a physical perspective. In the results, I also offer some suggestions about what to be considering next. It's one of my presents to you in the Fertile Foundations Toolkit.

So, what does it really take to make a baby? A healthy egg, a healthy sperm with enough velocity to penetrate the egg, and an accommodating womb, right? And if you have sex near the time of ovulation, these elements naturally find their way to each other and poof – you are either doomed or blessed depending on your perspective. Well, yes and no. These are some of the elements and one possible scenario, but there really is so much more to it than our eighth grade health class led us to believe.

We know that the main event of preparation, conception, and gestation happens in that magical place, the womb. This is the main venue and its architectural features are ground zero for whether or not this miraculous event can occur. What are we working with here? What is the quality of the uterine lining? Do we have endometriosis, PCOS, a uniquely shaped uterus, fibroids, or some other challenge?

The good news is most of these physical obstacles can be overcome either with traditional medical intervention or alternative treatments. In the end, we do not have to be defeated by these hurdles. Rather, we learn what we're dealing with, get clear on our treatment options, and proceed with confident choice.

The eggs and the sperm are the next two critical players. Regarding eggs, we want to understand what's happening at ovulation time in terms of how many are being made available and what condition they are in. There are ways to influence each of these aspects and I discuss them below. What I want you to know is that the age of your eggs (i.e. your age) and the timing in your cycle does not automatically equate to hope or doom. It's not that black and white, and you have the power to influence change here.

Sperm are funny little fellows, aren't they? In this case we want to understand what's happening at ejaculation in terms of how many sperm occur in a volume of semen, what percentage of those sperm are alive, how the living sperm move, and what shape they are. Although you can use an at-home sperm test, it will not give a complete picture. If you are looking for data, I recommend having a semen analysis performed by a fertility specialist. The good news is there are ways to influence the improvement of sperm quality and count.

Hormones are also critical players in the miracle of baby-making. In most cases, hormones can be influenced through environmental and nutritional interventions. Let's have a closer look at what that means.

Hormonal Harmony and Disharmony

Hormones are MVPs in the game of life. Our bodies naturally produce these powerful, sensitive, regulatory substances that influence the activity of our cells and organs. When our hormones are disrupted, every biochemical activity for life is affected – digestion, metabolism, growth, reproduction, and sleep cycles, for example.

The hormones we're most concerned with for fertility are thyroid hormones, estrogen, follicle stimulating hormone (FSH), luteinizing hormone (LH), progesterone, prolactin, adrenaline, cortisol, insulin, glucagon, and testosterone. Let's briefly look at how each one impacts fertility.

Thyroid Hormones

The thyroid hormones impact all of our cells and organs. If our body produces too much, our vital processes function too quickly. If our body produces too little, that function is too slow.

Thyroid hormones impact fertility specifically in how they regulate metabolism, promote fertility, support a healthy pregnancy, and grow a healthy baby. If you're challenged with putting on weight, releasing weight, or feel more tired more often than you think you should, I recommend having your thyroid levels checked. Although there are prescriptions to help regulate thyroid function, consider influencing thyroid function through nutrition and lifestyle first. This approach may be better for your fertility overall.

Estrogen

Estradiol is the most important one of the group of hormones referred to as "estrogen" when it comes to fertility, but all of them play their part. Estrogen influences the breasts, uterus, brain, bones, liver, heart, and other tissues.

The follicles release estrogen to build up the uterine lining. Estrogen not only helps to make a comfy place for baby to grow, it also prepares the fallopian tubes, cervix, and vagina to make everything receptive to incoming sperm.

Gonadotropins – Go, Go, Release the Eggs

Under optimal health conditions, the hypothalamus and the pituitary gland in the brain make the gonadotropins called follicle stimulating hormone (FSH) and luteinizing hormone (LH). Together they activate the release of the eggs or follicles by spiking at ovulation. They are also responsible for stimulating the production of estradiol and then progesterone at just the right time in a reproductive cycle to nurture the eggs to grow into babies.

Men's bodies produce FSH and LH too. For them, FSH and LH participate in controlling sperm and testosterone production. While FSH and LH can both be measured in blood or urine, LH is the one that gets measured when you pee on the stick of a home ovulation test.

Progesterone and Prolactin

Progesterone is produced by the ovaries and adrenal glands regularly, and also in the placenta during pregnancy. It influences sexual desire, helps regulate the menstrual cycle, helps the body prepare for pregnancy, and then supports and maintains pregnancy once the fertilized egg is nicely snuggled into the uterine lining. When pregnancy occurs, the elevated levels of progesterone and estrogen tell the ovaries not to release any more eggs, and help to grow the glands in the breasts that produce milk.

Prolactin is produced by the pituitary gland. In conjunction with progesterone, it helps to start and maintain the production of breast milk. Prolactin is present in men and women, but levels increase and stay high during the breastfeeding period in new mothers.

Adrenaline and Cortisol – Stress Hormones

Adrenaline and cortisol are produced by the adrenal glands, and are essential to biochemical balance across systems and tissues throughout the body. What's most important to understand is their relationship with stress. They influence blood sugar levels; muscle tension; the way the body uses fat, protein, and carbohydrates; immune system function, including inflammatory response; blood pressure; and the way the central nervous system responds to environmental stimuli.

The actions of adrenaline and cortisol are detrimentally pervasive in the way we live our lives today. Because they can have such a significant impact on fertility, it's important to understand the stress cycle as a beneficial natural occurrence, and how it's gone awry for most of us. Too much of a good thing is a bad thing.

As a species, we have inherited the "fight or flight" reaction to protect our ability to stay alive and make more humans. In the beginning, this mechanism was our friend – very pro procreation. For example, here's how it works *for* us to save us from the threat of a saber-tooth tiger. When a threat like the tiger is detected, cortisol activates the experience of fear, which impacts our mood and motivation, heightens our perception, and restricts or shuts down functions that are not essential or may be a hindrance during the need to take flight or engage in a defensive fight – this includes reproduction, digestion, immune response, and growth and development processes. Cortisol also increases the availability of substances used to repair body tissues in case of injury.

In collaboration with adrenaline, cortisol causes an accelerated release and use of glucose for an energy boost. Adrenaline supports physical readiness for action by increasing heart and breath rates, and increasing muscle tension. A mechanism that sets your body into action without you thinking about how to save your hide is great when you are under real threat.

When the threat is gone or resolved, our bodies go into a recovery, repair, and rest cycle in which the intensity of the hormones decreases, corresponding physical responses are deactivated, any physical damage is repaired, and suspended or diminished processes are re-activated.

Although we are not facing hot-blooded, live tigers in daily life, it is common for most of us to enter adulthood under the perpetual influence of stress. That means we are having a long-term experience of stress and all the reactive mechanisms described above. The cycle of recovery, repair, and rest is impaired.

The continuous exposure to high-levels of stress hormones becomes the body's new programming. Some of the undesirable outcomes include low energy, hypertension, digestive imbalances, decreased testosterone production, irregularity of the menstrual cycle, compromised immune system function, and slowed or diminished healing response. A brief list of possible stressors that we encounter on an average Tuesday might include workload, relationship conflict, financial concerns, heavy traffic, personal obligations, events in the news, and failed attempts at conception.

If you are experiencing any of the following on a regular basis, you are probably caught in a loop of long-term stress: tension, anxiety, nervousness, edginess, uncertainty, lack of focus, lack of control, hopelessness, helplessness, frustration, fear, headaches, indigestion, moodiness, or increased anger. These are some of the most common emotional states that people under constant stress experience at a very high frequency – so frequently, they may see a doctor about getting medication to manage the emotions. It's very common.

The Mayo Clinic says, "The subsequent overexposure to cortisol and other stress hormones, can disrupt almost all your body's processes." It is safe to say that these stressors, no matter their source, are the result of accepting stress-inducing thoughts that you have about a situation you find yourself in. For most of us, it just isn't true that our lives are under threat all day, every day. However, our emotional reaction to our thoughts can be very powerful in creating a long-term stress cycle.

Insulin and Glucagon

Insulin and glucagon work together to regulate blood sugar levels and keep them within a narrow range to provide a stable supply of energy. During some pregnancies, pregnancy hormones can cause disruption to the stability of the insulin-glucagon balance and result in gestational diabetes. Attention to nutrition is an important and effective way to support the sensitive collaboration of insulin and glucagon at any stage and especially during pregnancy.

Unstable blood sugar can trigger the immune system to produce an inflammatory reaction, increasing the need for more insulin. The increased inflammation leads to increased production of cortisol, which can inhibit other hormones important for healthy fertility. The inflammation also results in the swelling of tissues, resulting in impaired circulation.

Testosterone

Testosterone is produced in ovaries, testes, and adrenal glands. It triggers the manufacture of new blood cells, contributing to the strength of muscles and bones. It influences libido and the production of FSH and LH.

Low levels of testosterone in men can interfere with sperm production and quality. Overly high levels of testosterone in women can be disruptive to the ovaries.

Good Eggs

The ovaries are the home of the eggs till they are released at ovulation. During their time in the ovaries, their quality can be influenced by a woman's lifestyle. What she consumes, how much sleep she gets, and the impact on her chemistry from emotional events all impact egg quality. The important thing to understand is that this is all happening inside the ovaries – before the egg comes out to play in the field of conception.

It is clear the health of the ovaries determines the health of the eggs. However, there is much mystery around the origins and production of eggs that is still being discovered, and research in reproductive health continues at a heated pace. Stem cell research in conjunction with research in reproductive health indicates that we may form new eggs throughout what's referred to as the "reproductive years" – a term that may or may not have any real meaningful value.

What all this means for you is that ensuring overall health – physical, mental, and emotional – leads to enhanced fertility. Specifically, healthy ovaries need good blood flow and high-quality nourishment. Movement like massage and dance, belly laughs, and other physical activity increase blood flow to the pelvis. The blood is nourished by clean consumption – low- or non-toxic, non-aggravating foods and cosmetics. This blood flows to the ovaries, impacting the quality of the eggs stored there.

Care and Feeding of a Mom-to-Be

Are you aware that the biochemical foundation for a healthy conception begins at six months before the occurrence of conception? What does that mean? New cells began their development six months ago.

The collection of cells that is you today – the biochemical being you are today – was set into motion six or more months ago. What you are exposed to, what you eat, and what you think and feel today influences your overall composition of the future you six months down the road. It's on this foundation of composition that you try to conceive and carry your baby.

Your health is the foundation of your life. It truly impacts your experience in every moment – from what you think and feel to how you move and how you participate. When we are feeling frustrated and angry, stressed, helpless, or afraid to believe in anything, our health suffers. One of the first points of control for you regarding your fertility is your overall health. Grab this point of control and make the most of it. What do you need to change to create that healthy foundation? Sometimes we need help answering this question, but it's significantly worthwhile.

What does it mean to enter the baby-making process on a healthy foundation? It means it's time to get *you* into the best health that you can – because *you* is where this life will grow. Grow yourself into a vibrant garden of life force energy, and, out of this garden, grow your baby.

Nutrition is one of the vital pillars to fortify before going for motherhood. The good news is that it's the easiest, and the solutions are so accessible that there really is no reason to not check this box.

In the section Good Eggs, I referred to clean consumption: low- or non-toxic, non-aggravating foods and cosmetics. What does this mean?

Regarding food, we are talking nutrient-dense, non-toxic superfood and sensible, effective, and pure, superior-quality supplements. This will get you the best nutrition possible, feeding and nourishing those little eggs so they are happy and shiny, ready to make healthy babies when they come down the chute at ovulation.

Regarding cosmetics – from head to toe – there are many ways to check for the level of toxicity in a product. My favorite resources for checking out toxicity before I head for the check-out is the Environmental Working Group's Skin Deep Cosmetics Database. You can find it with a quick Google search. Search by brand, and if you can't find the products that way, search on the ingredients in the product for the toxicity of each element.

I leave the cosmetic research for my clients to do on their own. But I do have access to pure, superior-quality supplements and nutrient-dense, non-toxic superfood to share. Many women, myself and my clients included, have found that getting their bodies clean and then maintaining this level of "clean" brings a wealth of benefits, including enhanced fertility.

Beyond the Body

So far in this chapter we've been looking at the empirical half of the fertility equation. Now we shift to the other half of the picture. In my own struggles and then in my work with many others, I've seen how significant the impact of this other half truly is, despite its general underestimation.

When I was trying to become a mommy and the world seemed so very unfair, it didn't occur to me to get curious about what might be blocking my creative flow from an energetic perspective. I invite you to consider this question for yourself. A creative block is something that stands between you and what you want to create. In this case, I'm talking about a non-physical block – something of an energetic nature that has a significant density. It's the density of it that makes it a block – a heavy stuck thing, a thing standing between you and what you want to create – your baby. This is an obstacle that doctors cannot detect in lab results, and therefore they can't help you with it.

Even if you have some biochemically identified thing that must be managed so that baby-making can happen, wouldn't it be great to have the energetic thing already handled? So what might be blocking your creative flow? What stories are running in your head and influencing your body that could be contributing to your struggle or resistance? I'm referring to stories about pregnancy, delivery, motherhood, the parenting relationship, intimacy with your partner, and anything else that is part of the bigger picture of what it means to become a mommy.

How can you know what's contributing to your resistance? Check in with your body. It will tell you the truth every time.

Give yourself some time and space to do the investigation; have a notebook handy in case you want to take notes. If there's something that you felt a reaction to when you read the list of possible story topics above, that's a place to start. Otherwise, just pick one and try it on.

When you think about pregnancy, for example, what happens in your body? What body sensations do you experience? It may take some practice and you may need to try it out more than once to get reconnected with your body in this way, but my clients find the time they give it valuable, and what they learn from their own bodies very informative.

Notice and feel any body sensations as they come up when you are thinking about topics related to being a mommy. When you think about the labor and birthing process, what happens in your body? Do you experience a sense of blockage, gripping, heaviness, density, or darkness around certain aspects of motherhood?

I realize these ideas can be a bit esoteric or subtle, but tune into your body and open the conversation. You'll be surprised by what you can learn. I promise it's safe and there's nothing to fear here. This is about being openly curious with yourself.

If you encounter a blockage, notice the resistance. Get to know it in a sensory way. Sense into its qualities – sharp, hard, thin, wide, narrow, heavy, and so on. Be as curious as you can be and simply notice. Whatever you find, acknowledging its presence frees it up to go. You get to decide if this is a story that you want to keep, change, or let go of.

Once you sense the energy of a block and know it's there, you have the opportunity to transform it. The transformation will reopen your creative flow.

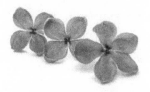

Chapter 4

Love and Hate in Your Most Important and Intimate Relationship

B efore I was in the thick of my fertility struggle, I had never considered the nature of the relationship between me, myself, and my body. What we're talking about here is the relationship that occurs in the intrapersonal realm. It involves the thoughts, and consequently the feelings you have about yourself. You've heard of self-talk; that's intrapersonal communication.

I wish someone had explained to me early on in my life that this is the most important and most intimate relationship I'll ever have. When you think about it, it seems so obvious, but it's not something that usually gets taught by parents or schools. While we get a lot of information about how to judge ourselves, we don't get a lot of information about how to appreciate and love ourselves, how to talk to ourselves, and how to support ourselves in growing into what we desire to become. What's relevant to our discussion here is how this intrapersonal relationship relates to becoming a mother.

Here's the flow of energy from thought to action or creation:

A thought in the mind → A feeling in the heart → Action or non-action in the body

The mind is where the self-talk happens, and in a nano-second flash, your heart or feeling-center is impacted. I refer to this collaboration as the heart-mind, and it's the most powerful source of creation or destruction in the Universe. You can think of this as the Holy Spirit, the Life Force, or energetic origin and essence. This mechanism is validated by spiritual traditions and modern scientific findings.

Are you beginning to see how the flow of energy from thought to creation impacts your movement from who you are now to the parent you want to become? Your desire to be a mommy is the heart-mind saying, "I want to be a mommy," and the creation is the baby. As you create the baby with body action, you become a different version of you – a parent. This is a huge deal for some of us. It's bigger than we were led to understand. And your only real partner on the intrapersonal level is you. You need you; you need your body to cooperate with you; you need your heart-mind to support you and your body in taking the actions that will result in your desired creation.

Three Possible Ways to Relate to Yourself

So what does your relationship with yourself look like right now? The three categories of possible ways to relate to yourself are:

A. You like or even love You

B. You dislike or even hate You

C. You are disconnected from and ambivalent about You

In scenario A, you have the most effective relationship for creating and experiencing what you want on both physical and metaphysical levels. You are your best ally, best friend, and best resource for moving through challenges. Even if it doesn't look perfect 100% of the time, you've got such a great advantage and a strong starting position. You may find that when you've faced challenges in the past, you are usually triumphant. The challenge you are facing now with your fertility is most likely about internal obstacles that you may or may not be aware of yet. You are still in the game, and with help opening the hidden doors, you can find your way out of this frustrating maze.

In scenario B, you are defeating yourself by criticizing, demoralizing, berating, threatening, and belittling yourself on a regular basis. No one feels good or motivated to cooperate with someone who treats them this way. You may notice that you struggle with a lot of things in your life. You may even notice that one of the reasons you want a baby is because of the fantasy of the kind of love and ease you feel when you picture the relationship between a mommy and a precious baby. You, like most of us, may be longing for unconditional love.

Do not take this as a hopeless message. In fact, reading this information may already be initiating a shift for you. The beginning of a shift is subtle, and you'll know it's happening because of the very faint sense of an opening that you haven't felt or sensed before. Even if it's not happening for you right now, I promise this shift is possible for you. It is possible for you to give yourself that unconditional love relationship you are longing to be a part of.

In scenario C, the disconnection and ambivalence are like a short circuit. You may live life solely from your head-space. Perhaps it's too painful to live from your body-space, or perhaps this is just the programming you've learned on your way to adulthood. When you have successes, most likely you either know the exact logic that delivered your success, or you are a bit surprised and unclear about how success actually happened. When you have challenges, you may prefer to find an easier path or give up the quest completely if you cannot foresee a clear and logical approach to the desired outcome. If your forward vision shows you a dead end or failure, you are likely to abandon the project.

The challenge you are facing now with your fertility may be the first time you're feeling moved to keep going despite the disappointment. You may be constantly wondering why you keep on; but this time your desire is bigger than your ambivalence – even when you think it doesn't really matter.

Whether you find yourself in scenario B or C, your programming has served you in some way in the past or you wouldn't be running this program at all. You can notice it and choose a different program going forward, but be patient with yourself and know that it takes time to implement the new program through consistent reconditioning. You always have a different choice. But first you have to become aware of it, and then you can choose.

Your Most Reliable Ally or Your Worst Enemy

By now you are either beginning to have a new understanding of your relationship with yourself, or you are newly aware that this relationship exists and is ultimately the most powerful influence in your life. You get to choose how you want to be treated and how you want to treat others. In this case, the others are yourself and your body. In effect, you get to choose how you want to relate to yourself.

You can be your most reliable ally or your worst enemy. What will it be? If you are to overcome the obstacles between you and motherhood, begin here. There is healing to be done. The progression of healing begins with establishing that connection – the relationship. If you find yourself in scenario C, this is Step 1: Connect.

Even if your relationship with yourself and your body is adversarial, as in scenario B, begin with simply appreciating that you have the relationship. In time, this relationship can be your superpower instead of your kryptonite. Right now, it is the framework of your healing space and now is your healing time.

Take a deep breath; walk forward toward yourself. It's time to get vulnerable and raw with some self-investigation. You may find that you want some outside support for the next steps.

Good Intentions Gone Awry

As you try to conceive over a period of time without success or with loss, you will understandably encounter stress related to these events, month after month. When do you have time for recovery, repair, and rest? On top of the stress related to the unsuccessful pursuit of motherhood, you may have already been experiencing accumulated stress during your life without recovery or downtime.

I am writing these words as if I am speaking to you while looking at you with love in my eyes. Please read them that way. Remember what you are wanting to create. Remember what you are asking your body to do – create life. How are you going about this? And so we begin the self-investigation.

Are you packing your life full of obligations that don't ultimately have to be yours? Are you going to baby showers that are painful to attend? Are you staying up late reading or watching everything you can that might inform you about the best way to get pregnant – including this book? Are you burning the candle at both ends without taking breaks to move your body and feed it well?

Are you thrashing away at your body with medical treatments and a mercenary search for that elusive answer somewhere outside of yourself? Are you keeping yourself distracted from your uncomfortable feelings with food and drink, entertainment, other busy occupations and overstimulation? Does it feel like you're holding your breath a lot of the time? How are you holding your face and your body – relaxed or tense?

Be aware of what you are intending with these pursuits. You may have set up a framework of busy-ness and effortful pursuit of being a good person and running toward the next thing that might get you to the promised land of motherhood. This behavior may arise from "good intentions," but it will ultimately defeat you.

You will be better served by taking a step back to see the whole picture instead of being in the thick of this forest. As you back up and get the wider perspective, I encourage you be thorough and take a slower pace, deeper breaths, and engage your heart-mind to know, be, and do what will really move you forward.

Operator, Can You Please Connect Me?

The connection you have with yourself is the most powerful resource within your reach. There is a lot of information available in our popular culture about compassion for yourself and self-acceptance. But how much have you engaged with these notions? Have you decided that soft stuff is for someone else? Do you consider it weak-minded, selfish, or self-indulgent? I promise you it's the strongest most generous place to start.

I assure you this connection is vital for you always and especially right now. Here's an exercise to dip your toe in and learn something more about your relationship with yourself. For one whole week, notice – without making any changes – how you talk to yourself in your head and how you talk about yourself to others. What kinds of words do you use about yourself or your actions when you are telling a friend or co-worker about something you did? What is the tone of the voice that speaks to you in your head, commenting on what you are doing and how you are doing it? Do you ever look at yourself in the mirror and really see yourself? What does that voice in your head say about what you see in the mirror?

If you heard someone saying these things in this way about your dear friend or your child, would you be okay with it? Is that how you would talk to them yourself? If your answer is "no" to either of these questions, I invite you to decide right now that this type of self-talk is no longer acceptable. It's time to begin loving yourself – first with your thoughts and words, and then your loving actions will naturally follow.

Biggest Needs Right Now

As you become more loving toward yourself, your connection with yourself will grow stronger. You'll be more able to respond to your own needs, and then you can effectively understand and alleviate the continuous stress cycle that you are currently experiencing. When you can rely on yourself to take care of you and your body beyond daily personal hygiene, you are ready to take on your stress monster.

First look at what is causing your stress and how you can impact that cause. How do you react to those things that you've identified as stressors? You may not be able to control a situation, but you can choose your reaction to it. Choosing a different, less stressful reaction to common situations that trigger you is where you begin.

Even better, if you can take control of the stress-creating situations, do that. In practical application, this action might look like modifying schedules and commitments. Consider what's necessary, what's "nice" to have or do, and what's irrelevant. Remove your attendance at irrelevant situations. Choose discerningly what "nice" to have or do situations you will be available to. Arrange the necessary situations to the extent of your influence so that they serve and support you when possible.

Next look at how you are caring for yourself physically. How might you modify your nourishment, either in quality or quantity? There are foods you want to avoid and foods you want to consume that can support your pursuit of parenthood.

Your body is made to move. Movement activates endorphins. Endorphins make you feel good. What kind of movement activity did you enjoy when you were little? Here are a few suggestions: bicycling, dancing, swimming. Find a way to move more than just from the car to the house, to the couch, to the bed.

On the flip side, if you're an obsessive marathoner or gym rat, see what happens when you try something gentler, less intense, something that feels soft and nurturing – like a solo slow dance. There are so many ways to fulfill the basic body need of movement, there really is no excuse not to meet this need. Make it a non-negotiable, like you do with brushing your teeth.

Allow your body to rest. This may sound too simple, but it is deeply profound. Do you get enough sleep? And what is the quality of that sleep? There are many factors that can influence your ability to get into a restorative sleep state and maintain it for a long enough period of time. To start with, consider that sleep is an act of surrender. As you fall asleep, you surrender your waking consciousness. It's an act of faith to let go of the day and move into the unknown. It's a valuable practice with a daily opportunity.

Allow the mattress to hold you; fall into its support. Feel the sheets below and above you. Feel the pillow under your head. Fall. Release your physical self to be held by the bed. Give your mind a place to anchor till it can float on the space of the dream state. An anchor that works well for me and many of my clients is the breath. Notice where your breath is in your body, and see if you can ease it into an ebb and flow that reaches more parts of your body and carries you off to the land of nod.

Another practice that can be supportive to nighttime surrender is journaling. Empty your mind onto the page before you lay your head down to rest. Let the notebook catch and hold all your thoughts or lists for tomorrow and all the mental residue from today. It will all be there in the morning if you want to pick it up again.

The process of surrendering into sleep not only supports you from a physical relaxation standpoint, but also supports your emotional health. The practice of intentional relaxation is a practice of controlling the mind which eases the emotions.

During the day, put your energy into the relationships that support you. With those that you trust the most, let them know what you're going through, and be as clear as you can be about what you need from them right now. It may be a request for them to understand why you're less available or how you need to talk about what you're going through without having them offer a solution. You may just want some empathy; you can request that.

Find ways to be amused. How can you look at situations that you find yourself in and see some humor? Choose experiences that make you smile and laugh – including funny movies or books or friends. And of course, get the professional help you need when you see that you need it. All of these suggestions are strong antidotes for the healthy reduction and management of stress, and all of them enhance your body's functions – including fertility.

Part 3

BROKEN HEART-MIND

"What is the knocking at the door in the night?
It is somebody wants to do us harm.
No, no, it is the three strange angels.
Admit them, admit them."

– D. H. Lawrence

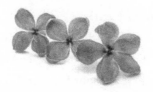

Chapter 5
The C Word

The C word ... what could that be? I am referring to "commitment." According to the *Oxford English Dictionary*, commitment is "the state or quality of being dedicated to a cause, or activity, such as a pledge, undertaking, engagement or obligation that restricts freedom of action." We'll use this definition to guide us as we explore how commitment applies to fertility.

Are You Crazy Enough to Be Committed?

Becoming a parent is a big commitment. It can be daunting, especially if you're a high-achiever who tends toward perfectionism. Once we are moving toward parenthood and actively doing the do to make the baby, we assume we are committed to the process and the outcome. What if this is a false assumption? What if you are in a place of muddle? How do you know if you're committed, and if you find you're not, how do you become and stay committed? After all, how will you see it through without commitment?

I find the last few words in the above definition of commitment to be very interesting. That part about an engagement that restricts freedom of action. The message here is about focus and clarity of vision. Do you have a clear vision of yourself as a parent? Have you fully resolved any conflict that could hold you back from confidently moving forward? Has the strength of your desire to become a mom quashed any other possibility for your future?

On a scale from 0 to 10, 0 being "no way" and 10 being "no matter what," where does your level of commitment land? There is no judgment to execute here, but there is valuable information to discover. I am doubtful there's anyone reading this book – other than my curious friends and family, maybe – who would land at the 0 end of the scale. However, if you are between 5 and 7, it's time to step back from the baby-making pursuit and get real with yourself. Do you really want a baby? Is there a quality about the experience of motherhood that you are looking for, longing for, that you can get to without a baby?

You may be feeling very conflicted about whether or not you want to be a mom, and there's nothing wrong with being unsure. However, pushing yourself forward reluctantly is not the way to go. I promise it's not good for you or your partner. You are living in a mixed message to yourself, to your body, to your partner, and to the waiting spirit of the incoming baby.

I've spoken to many women who were not sure that being a mom was something they had always dreamed of or wanted. One woman, we'll call her Anna, told me that although she'd been trying for more than three years, she wasn't really sure she wanted to be a mom. She was trying because if *maybe* she and her partner wanted to be parents someday, biologically now was the time. In the next breath she told me that she was trying to believe that she still had time and didn't really have to decide just yet. So on one hand she was pushing herself based on time urgency, and on the other hand there was no rush. The only part of that message that was clear was that she was in conflict.

Ultimately, when she was ready to get really honest, we were able to discover that she was holding back a lot of emotion. Until she allowed that emotion to come through and process, she couldn't really know what she wanted. Our work together was mainly about exploring that muddle and bringing her fears and her options out into the light. This was hard work for her – she didn't even want to think about it, never mind feel the feelings, but she knew she needed to face it in order to stop the torture of the conflict.

Your Space-Time Container

Let's go back to the "Are you committed to becoming a mommy" scale and the idea that commitment implies focus and clarity of vision. Let's say you're somewhere between 8 and 10 on the scale. That sounds like a solid commitment, and it certainly is a stronger place to start from than 7 or less. Good to go, right? Well, if you're struggling, I'd say this is still a place to check out.

Let's look at the arrangement of your life. What does your space-time container look like? Do you have space and time for a child in your life?

What is the environment that you're currently living in? Can you picture your child living there with you? When you look around, do you know where your little one's stuff will go in this living arrangement, or do you have plans to move?

Do you have time in your life for a child? It could be as simple a solution as your plan to change the way you spend your time once you're a mom. But if you've never thought about it before, do the exercise now.

It can be surprising to learn that you haven't actually considered where your baby fits into the time and space of your life. I was working with a client, we'll call her Chelsea, who was very distraught about not conceiving after trying with dedication and assistance for almost four years. She was a very hard worker in every area of her life and was able to create a lot of success for herself. She understood commitment. However, during one of our sessions I asked her to describe in detail what her life would look like five years down the road. I encouraged her to let her imagination run wild.

Her answer surprised both of us. She described the new qualifications she would achieve from further education and her new role in her career. She talked about where she and her husband would be living, how much money they would be making, and the travel they would be doing. What she never mentioned in her description was a child. Her vision did not include one.

Chelsea was in shock at this discovery. It literally took her breath away. And so we began designing a new vision for her, one aligned with her deep-heart longing for a baby.

I share this story to highlight how we sometimes unknowingly make assumptions that result in tricky undoing. This is something no urine or blood test can reveal. I invite you to investigate the vision you are holding for your future. Picture that baby involved in your daily circumstances if that's what you want. In a situation like this, if we can't see it happening, it can't happen. Our desire and our vision must be aligned.

The Art of Creation

Getting to parenthood is an act of creation – this is art and science coming together in a beautiful dance. I encourage you to approach it from this angle. Use your written, spoken, and thought language to support this creation. Choose your activities discerningly in support and service of this creation. Not only are you architecting new life in the form of a baby, but you are also evolving the present version of you into who you are becoming in the form of a mommy. Allow for conception, gestation, and birth of you into parenthood, and baby into life.

This is a perfect time to look at how you relate to yourself and others. We covered your relationship with yourself in the last chapter. Here I want to briefly look at how we relate to others, specifically around our responsibility to them. Sometimes we have a pattern of doing too much for others. It's time to release responsibility to its rightful owner.

Another trend that I see in women like us who struggle with fertility is a pattern of wanting to take care of everything and everybody. We overwhelm ourselves with obligations of our own making. We hate to say "no" when someone asks us for something. There's generosity and then there's self-sacrifice, not in a good way. When generosity and self-sacrifice hurt you and get in the way of what you want to create in your own life, it's time for some reconditioning.

You are not responsible for other people's feelings, suffering, emotional well-being, successes, or failures. You are not here to fix people or their situations. Rather we can practice empowering others so they can do for themselves. You are important. and I'm sure you are contributing to the lives of your loved ones and others every day. However, if you checked out for a week, I promise the world would not fall apart. If you give them a chance, people who are used to relying on you to fix them or their situations can figure it out for themselves. We are free to release these responsibilities. When we choose to empower others, it not only helps us, but it elevates them too.

Also notice where your mothering energies are going right now. Who or what is taking up the time and space that your child will occupy?

As you notice and release through letting go or delegation, you will feel a shift, an opening, a moment of concern quickly followed by relief. As if an unseen window has been opened in front of you, you will feel a rush of fresh air and lightness. Do this for yourself. Do this for your baby. This is one powerful way you can make room in your space and time for you and your baby to come into being together as parent and child.

Choosing Commitment

Do you ever feel that life happens to you, signs you up for things you didn't freely agree to? Sometimes we can feel like our level of commitment just happens to us; and it will, indeed, unless we consciously claim our intentions. Again we are talking about focus and clarity of vision. You get to decide what you are committed to.

What do you want in your life? What are your intentions?

If this is new for you, I want you to know that you get to choose. There is no "should" here in any direction. The field is wide open, and all the elements are at our disposal. What do you commit to? What are you willing to do and where do you draw the line? It's equally valuable to know what you're *not* willing to do. This equally contributes to defining your commitment.

Throughout this chapter we've explored commitment and its relationship to relieving the struggle women like us experience on the way to motherhood. It is infinitely valuable to understand yourself, know what you're unclear and muddled about, and then take a time-out while you get clear and define what you want to commit to so that you can confidently continue your journey toward parenthood. This single exercise can relieve struggles of all kinds.

No Commitment Without Clarity

Before you can get to that ease and relief, there has to be the clearing away, a closet cleaning if you will, of junk that you've been storing in the dark. We often keep this stuff in storage because it may have served to protect us in the past. But now, this stuff is in the way, blocking creative flow and maintaining the muddle.

Becoming a parent is huge and life-changing. Because we recognize that, it's part of the reason we struggle. It's time to clean out the closet and unpack these concerns. Doing so can free you to really embrace clarity and move forward from commitment.

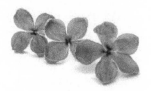

Chapter 6
Out of the Closet

N ow that we've pulled those hidden concerns out of the closet, let's unpack them together. This is the part of the process where you get familiar with where you're coming from. By understanding the thought patterns that you've relied on up to this point in your life, you can understand what's not working for you anymore. This is also a great opportunity to question what's really true, what you want to keep, and what you want to replace. Let's shine the light on the beliefs that have been running the show.

Waiting for Perfect

Remember those standards and values we grew up with that told us it was irresponsible to get pregnant if you didn't have the right relationship, home, and financial stability in place first? These were instilled in us with the best of intentions. Consequently, we spent years holding up barriers to pregnancy with our thoughts, plans, pills, condoms, gels, sponges, creams, and such. All of this had our focus trained like a laser on prevention. It's like a force field.

Now that we're here at the place of wanting a baby and not getting the desired result, it makes sense to question what we really mean by these parameters – the right time, place, financial situation, and relationship. I suggest that if a quest for the perfect alignment of these pieces is what you've been concerned about or waiting for on any level at all, you are on an endless quest. There is no destination on that journey. There truly will never be a perfect alignment of all these elements.

There is no certainty to find in that search. Where you can find certainty is within your heart-mind desire. I'm repeating myself here because it's so important: Your heart gives you a desire not to torture you, but to lead you in the direction of fulfilling the promises of your life. Your soul is speaking to you.

If concerns about having these elements in place just so looms large for you, let's acknowledge that. Don't stuff them back into the dark. Take a moment to allow them to be present; really consider what the concerns have to tell you about changes you may want to make so that you can confidently get on with fulfilling the potential of your life.

I promise you this is about much more than having a baby. There are important messages for you to receive from these concerns. For example, if you're in a relationship that you believe is not good to bring a baby into, I encourage you to consider whether or not it's a good relationship for you to stay in.

Relationship Remodel

A very common concern is how the arrival of a baby will impact your relationship with your significant other. It was one of my biggest concerns. I really enjoyed having my husband to myself, and I was loving the life we were creating together.

There's much research on how becoming parents changes a couple's dynamics. You may want to give some of that research a read if you're really curious. Most of us make our way through the transition from childless couple to parents either based on or in contrast to what was modeled for us by our parents.

It's true that your primary relationship will change. You can think of evolving into parenthood as the dawning of version 2.0 of your couplehood. Be open, be flexible, stay vulnerable, and practice intentional communication from that open, flexible, vulnerable state. That's all I'll say on the evolution for now, or we'll be entering into a different book.

It is true that the relationship you have with your significant other is a very important component of your life. If you're reading this book, you've most likely been committed to your relationship with this person for more than two years, and you may have been together much longer.

Are you in agreement that you both want to become parents? If there is any doubt on either side, it's worth exploring together with the help of a neutral third party. Sometimes it's hard to know what questions to ask and sometimes it's hard to hear a question from a significant other in the neutral way we can hear it from a third party.

I'll continue here with the assumption that you are both open to becoming parents. Once you're in agreement, you may find that the process of trying to conceive is now trying your relationship. Things get awkward when sex is no longer spontaneous and the definition of "satisfied" means the presence of double lines or a plus sign on a stick you peed on.

If you've become obsessed with your path to motherhood, then conversations with your significant other are also probably not what they used to be. It's no longer fun; in fact, it's strained. Your partner may be afraid to touch you except when it's show time. Your partner may also fear saying the wrong thing and upsetting you. Strained conversation leads to limited communication. That's when you begin to experience feelings of overwhelm and isolation of making decisions on your own.

You don't want to let your partner down, and your partner just wants to take care of you and support you. As you may be experiencing, difficulty with fertility generally creates added stress on a relationship. Sometimes it's hard for each of you to have a shared understanding of what's going on, what the real choices are, and where you want to put your money and your faith. It's frustrating to say the least.

I worked with a couple who, during their pursuit of parenthood, had been very diligently trying all different approaches for about four years. At the point that I met them, their biggest challenge was getting on the same page. Sara and Luke never seemed to be at the same conclusion point for the next best step forward. It was difficult for them to be open with and mutually supportive of each other for fear of setting the other off. They each felt it was safer to keep a distance.

Ultimately, their way of coping was to shut down from each other. They felt stuck and didn't know what to do next. They felt overwhelmed by all of the choices and had little confidence or preference for any of the options. They felt inhibited by the high costs and low success rates of solutions offered to them.

Through our sessions together, I guided their communication with questions that allowed them each safe space to open up and express what was in their hearts. We made agreements about how our sessions would work at the outset, and then we dove in. The goal was to bring them together in safe, vulnerable communication, and to experience collaboration.

They each gained better insight about where their partner was emotionally in the wholeness of their lives, not just in the area of making a baby. Information about how each of them felt about their own parents and childhood was shared. Sara mentioned that she appreciated seeing Luke reveal himself in a way that wasn't happening in daily life.

As our time together ended, the tone of their relationship had shifted. There was a softening and slowing down, a releasing of the urgency to get to the "magic treatment" already. I am happy to report that Sara and Luke have been able to move forward together more closely with some tools to keep the fun in their relationship and the sense of "us" that they had lost for a time.

Career Fears

A lot of women, me included, have legitimate concerns about the impact motherhood will have on their careers. At the very least, career women will have a time-out when it's labor and delivery time and after baby arrives. This hiatus does not have to be long. And it does not have to be short. Once again, you get to choose.

Sometimes we make plans to either go back to work in a short period of time or stay home longer with the baby; and then we may find that the reality of the choice we made while we were pregnant does not suit us. It really can go either way, and it's truly hard to predict. It may be a universal hardship to the heart to separate from baby in those early days back to work, but what follows is unforeseeable.

And let's be clear this is not the real meat of the matter that might be holding you back from your successful pursuit of motherhood. No. What's more pertinent is that your experience of your career is going to change. No matter what you choose, it's going to change in some way, and how exactly it will change is ultimately unknowable until you're there.

Is this something you're allowing to get in the way? Are you holding this concern above your desire to be a mom? There are no rights or wrongs; there are just things to notice and different choices to make.

Money Mayhem

I've said before, and here it is again: When baby comes home, things change. If you are reading this section, I'll assume that your access to money is not unlimited. It is true that your standard of living can be significantly impacted by the expansion of your family. And here we are at another place of choice. You get to choose how you will use your money. Based on values that you and your significant other share, I encourage you to design your own standard of living that works in your financial framework.

Typically, financial concerns are another form of blockade we've been holding up against the "threat" of early pregnancy. When we arrive at the river ready to cross over to motherhood, this deeply ingrained pattern of blockage may steadfastly be continuing to do its original job.

To know whether this is part of what's contributing to your struggle, notice how you talk about money and the expenses related to getting pregnant and then bringing home baby. The language you're using tells your internal story right out loud.

If you notice that your story is about how you can't afford treatments or time off or fun anymore, notice how this contributes to the message of "No" when you are asking the question of whether now is the right time to have a baby. You can let this be the focus of your struggle; many of us do. Or you can know that you have defined spending limits that you are comfortable with, that you adhere to without blaming those choices for why you're not a mom.

What often happens is that we attach our disappointment and anger to the topic of money and how it shows up (or doesn't show up) in our life. But whether or not you become a mom is not about the money. What's more relevant here is that it's convenient to use money as a place to put your focus; it looks good from the outside to be responsibly concerned about money. However, this may just be a distraction from your internal conflict about becoming a mom.

The way to understand if this concern is serving only to keep you from working through your conflict about becoming a mom is to look at where you'd be if you took money completely out of the equation. In other words, ask yourself, "If I had a reliable source of income to cover my monthly expenses ten times over, would I still be conflicted around having a baby?"

As long as we're not clear, not committed to becoming a mom, we are in conflict. We send ourselves and our bodies a mixed message, and we will continue to get mixed results.

The first step here is to get clear about whether or not you are still in conflict about motherhood. If that's the case, all these other concerns are a smoke screen. Looking at them, trying to resolve them, will not get you different results. Different results come once we resolve the real conflict. And we must not be fooled into thinking we've got the "to be or not to be a mother" conflict resolved if it's really not. If there's a feeling of tension as you read this, now is a good time to go back and read Chapter 5 – The C Word, again.

Age Old Traditions Anew

A question of ongoing debate from both medical and moral perspectives is what age is too old to have a baby. How do we resolve this question once and for all? This boils down to your individual biological capacity coupled with your desire to be a mother. If your deep-heart desire drives you to fulfill this soul request, then wherever you are on the spectrum, from regularly ovulating to opting for IVF with donated eggs, you are not too old to be a mom. That's my take. You get to decide what's true for you. Whatever you believe, that's what's true.

There are many naysayers regarding the quest for motherhood beyond the late 30s. I'm not interested in reiterating those arguments here. I want to look you in the eyes with love and say, "Your heart knows your truth. Let that be your guide."

In our exploration throughout this chapter, we are sleuthing what might be standing between you and your baby – what is feeding your struggle. Age can be one of those sticky contributors. We are continually evolving. The average age of a new mother is all over the map now. According to the CDC, the mean age for mothers at first births is on the rise as a general trend. I have personally observed a wide range among mothers in my son's age group. As I write this, he is in the first grade, and his peers at school and in activities outside of school have moms ranging from their late 20s to their early 50s. That is a very broad range.

What does age mean for you in relation to your opportunity to be a mother? Is it simply a biological determinant, or is there more? Continuous and rapid progress in advanced reproductive technology are making what seemed impossible ten years ago possible today.

Again, it's time to ask if you are making this an overly burdensome concern and moving your focus away from other fears or concerns about becoming a mother. This one is stickier and more twisted than matters of money, career, or relationship. Your age and your biology are interconnected – and we are now capable of sustaining our biological capacities for longer than we ever were before.

In the area of age concerns, it's often useful to consider how well you care for yourself. How healthy are you now and how healthy can you be going forward for as long as your child is reliant on you? This of course involves making projections into uncertainty. But you already know what choices you are making and how they are impacting your health. Will that trajectory of patterned behavior continue? If not, how will it change and when? If you want to be a mom, what is going to support your best physical state to be there for your child to the degree that it's within your control?

If age is a real issue for you, address it so that you can clear it out of the way and get to any other underlying factors aggravating your journey to parenthood. Age is one of those surface issues. Most of us need some support with this one, but be gentle with yourself. You have the courage. Consider age from the frame of how you are as a whole person at this age rather than a pre-defined "norm." Understand the facts you're working with, and then make empowered decisions. And as with each of these suggestions, get help for the investigation and reflection processes when you need it.

My Unfinished List

But what about all the great things you wanted to accomplish before your freedom would be compromised by motherhood? If this is a big obstacle for you, know that I and a large group of other women are standing right beside you.

It's true that once you're a mom, you are probably going to be less likely to pack a sack and hike out to the wilderness. You're also less likely to jet off to New York for the weekend with girlfriends. With baby on board, there will be more planning involved for any adventure, even when you bring baby along. As my mom likes to say, "Life is a trade-off. Make your choice." There are no wrong choices; just different outcomes.

If you haven't already done this exercise, now is a great time. Make a list, you can call it a Bucket List if you want, of all the things you thought or dreamed you would have accomplished in your life by now or that you want to accomplish before you die. Review your list to see if any of the items are restricted by time (like you need to do it before someone dies or stops offering the event), money (that you need to accumulate first), or age (those bouncy houses for kiddos seven and under).

With this clear picture of all the things you want to do – they are captured and you can add to the list as you discover more – you can decide if you're going to let them get in the way of being a mother or not. You get to decide if something on your list is for you to do or work toward now or later. There is time for everything that you're actually going to do in your life, whatever that includes or excludes. Is being a mother on your list? Is that something for now or for later?

Good Enough Mother

Can you be the perfect mother you've always imagined? The reality is no one can. What we can be is the good enough mother – the mother that we wanted and who lives a real life. Let's lay this to rest right here if we can, because this concern is prohibitive for many of us. It almost paralyzed me, and it's a popular topic with my clients.

Generally speaking, you'll start out as a new mom tending to your new baby's needs as completely as is humanly possible. As the days go by, your ability to attend to every need will diminish by nature. It actually serves the kiddo to understand that Mom doesn't "fix" everything. And from a kid's point of view, every parent fails at meeting all the child's needs. Go easy on yourself here. There's an entire psychological theory of the Good Enough Mother developed by psychoanalyst and pediatrician Donald Winnicott in the early 1950s. It's for real.

If you have the capacity to be a loving person, you will be a loving mother. You, just like the rest of us, will have really hard days and you'll do the best you can. Every mom in the history of the world has never been the perfect mom. Not every mom, but most, can be the good enough mom, and that's what every kid needs. I'll bet that's you and me.

The crux of the matter for all of the concerns discussed in this chapter is the uncomfortableness of uncertainty. Each one of these common concerns haunts us from the halls of the unknown. There is no knowing exactly how the journey toward parenthood will pan out for you. And whatever you think you've nailed down right now, it is not guaranteed tomorrow. There is much here that requires your faith and your confidence in knowing what your standards and values are, because they will drive you to act in certain ways. That's what you are committed to consciously or unconsciously.

There are many life experiences that drop us into the deep end of the pool of uncertainty, and parenthood is one of the most uncertain of all. You see, there's an unknown person involved here and many other uncontrollable and even unforeseeable variables. The extent of your control of this situation is extremely limited. However, the extent of your control of your response to the situation is infinitely unlimited.

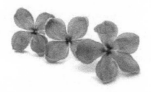

Chapter 7

Other Residue Hiding Just Beneath Your Skin

And now, my darling, we have to look at some difficult stuff. But I've got you. Let's get to the residue that's affecting our fertility like a ubiquitous and powerful infection. It interferes with our clarity of intention. This residue is made up of the fears and unconscious habits that we haven't addressed yet. I've alluded to them as we've gone along, but here we're going to get right to the nitty gritty. In Chapter 6, we made our way through some very common concerns that underlie what we'll look at next.

Lessons About Motherhood

Were you the little girl who carried a knowing in her heart that one day she would be a mommy? There was no question about it; it was a given. Or were you the little girl who didn't have any mothering inclinations whatsoever? This compulsion you feel now and that is causing disruption in your life may be relatively new for you. Either way, what you learned about being a mom as you grew up and that has developed through your family lineage is now in full fruition.

The legacy of motherhood that we inherit via family, popular culture, and our experience with the moms we knew while growing up have all informed our concept of "mom" – who she is and what it means to be her. These impressions that we unconsciously carry with us can contribute to that deep conflict and ambivalence about becoming a mother. Unearthing what's there and releasing it frees us up to define ourselves as the mother that we want to become.

There are a lot of sources of influence, so where do we start when we want to really understand what's got a hold of us? The best place is right at home.

What did you learn about motherhood and parenting from your family? And how does that information feel in your body?

For example, Jacqui, who was 38 when she came to me, was wrestling with the conflict of feeling pulled toward motherhood and repelled at the same time, like many of my clients. It was very confusing and disconcerting. She tried to ignore the conflict and decided to try to conceive – and this was her scenario for about three years. She pushed herself forward and acted as if she was clear. But the thing is, the truth still exists even when we ignore it.

In our work together we explored what she had learned about mothering when she was growing up. Her mother was a hardworking, independent woman with high standards who, despite her insecurities and self-esteem challenges, made decisions that moved her and her daughter from very humble beginnings to a more expansive lifestyle. In doing so, Jacqui often felt that her needs were a second priority.

She wanted more attention from her mother, more time with her mother; she wanted to be able to share the bad and the ugly of her life experiences with her mother, not just the good and pretty ones. Jacqui learned that mothers are really not available, and that her fantasy of what a good mother would be was simply that – a fantasy. Her fear was that there was no other way a woman could be a mom despite the woman's best intentions to be as available to the child as her child could want. And maybe a busy mother who was keeping it all together and maintaining high standards just couldn't possibly be available for what was not good and pretty – after all, bad and ugly does not meet high standards.

And then there was Jacqui's grandmother. She was hardworking in the home where Jacqui's mother grew up. This strong mother figure cared for her demanding husband and five kids, whose ages spanned a ten-year range. To Jacqui, her grandmother always looked exhausted, busy, and generally unavailable. She got the practical needs taken care of – everyone was always fed, clothed, and the house was tidy, but there wasn't time for softer moments of connection with lingering hugs or long conversations with eye contact over a cup of cocoa.

Jacqui acutely felt the absence of space for sharing humanity with both these women. It felt like they were just beyond reach. Jacqui also strongly desired to not create this feeling or this type of relationship with her own children, if she would have any someday.

The way Jacqui's grandmother and mother demonstrated motherhood left an uneasy, disappointed, sick feeling in her at the top of her stomach just below where her ribs come together. As she tapped into this body sensation in connection to her notions about how motherhood had disappointingly been modeled for her, she was struck by how strongly her own sense of personal power was impacted. She noticed that it was affecting how she expressed herself in her work, in her relationships, and in the way she managed money and made financial decisions.

The most beautiful realization was that Jacqui could choose something different for herself not only in each of these areas of her life, but also in how she wanted to be a mother. She described it like the feeling of a large rising air bubble, that once she found it there inside, it was loosened and dislodged. It rose up like a big, uncomfortable burp that she let out. With it, a pressure she hadn't previously been fully aware of was also defused. Coming to this awareness changed Jacqui's life in a powerfully positive way.

What have you learned about motherhood and how has that informed your picture of what's possible for you? I invite you to think about this question and feel into the answers. It's helpful to look directly at models of motherhood that were most prevalent in your life growing up – especially before the age of five. These have the deepest impact. As you make discoveries of what's lodged inside you and where, take the next step of thanking it for the information, and then choosing how you want to define the possibility of motherhood for yourself.

What You Don't Know Awaits

Entering into pregnancy and then motherhood are movements of action plus faith. You show up, do your part, and then wait and watch and respond to what evolves in response to your actions, feelings, and thoughts. By now you understand that your thoughts – the ones you are aware of and the ones that slip by unnoticed – are powerful influences creating your feeling state, which drives your actions. You are always moving toward a target based on what your mind produces. Real power comes with growing more aware of what your mind is producing. Taking the role of self-influencer to redirect your mind and consequently manage your emotions is an empowering reconditioning process. With this process, you have the power to influence your fertility journey.

The whole conception-to-parenthood passage can be fraught with the fear of entering the unknown. It involves a certain surrendering to a process of experience, a large portion of which is beyond your control. We can move into and through this venture with more power and comfort by literally letting go of and being ok with the part that we cannot influence, and then focusing on the part that we can.

You are contemplating making a separate individual who you ultimately cannot completely manage. As your little one moves out into the world, your ability to manage her experience and choices diminishes. This is the way it's supposed to be; this is healthy human development.

No-Joy Zone

Getting pregnant and becoming a mom is serious business, right? Well, it can be, and it can alternatively be joyous business at the same time. There are a range of ways to experience this journey, and if you haven't guessed by now, I'm of the belief that there can be ease even in the face of pain. This is a unique adventure with unforeseeable terrain that you will cross one way or another.

It's important to feel the excitement, joy, trepidation, fear, anticipation, grief – all the emotions – not only on this journey but in every life experience. You are a whole person with a whole life. You are more than your fertility. You are more than your miscarriages. You are more than your losses. And you are more than your wins. You are a whole person with a whole life, so I want to encourage you to keep expanding into your wholeness in those moments that might trigger you to contract into a small aspect of your larger life.

Anything you're involved in can be serious business, and being able to assess what attitude and mindset will best support your desired outcome is an important skill. When we can identify what will enhance the outcome we want, we can choose the attitude and mindset to adopt. This is a power move and you have the power to move this way. If this skill is new to you, be assured you can learn it.

Because the very nature of becoming a mom is a creative act, there is a natural contribution to be made by joy and love in this creation. Keeping out the light keeps the seeds of potential underground. Find ways to engage in what makes you smile. Yes, feel the other less pleasant emotions; and remember to actively lift yourself with opportunities to feel loved, to feel fun, to feel beautiful. These very opportunities contribute to the fullness and health of your fertility. Moving into the dark and staying there is a move of collapse. It happens to all of us.

Before you go for your next fertility treatment, prepare yourself and your body for the best potential of success. And if you're in the middle of a treatment process, do it now. Find the window where the light comes in and stand in the rays.

This is one of those actions on our behalf that we usually need help with. After all, if we could magically make ourselves feel better, wouldn't we be feeling better? Yes, and no; it is ultimately in your power, but we need each other, especially in times like these. Let someone you trust know that you need help; let them know you need them to help you get back into the light. Remember the things that make you smile and laugh; do those things with a trusted friend.

So Much Noise

As you survey the landscape of the fertility conversation, you may notice there's a lot of noise. The noise is divergent and discordant. And there's a lot of rubbish noise about "infertility" – it's so painfully common. Have you been talked into it yet? Have you been convinced that there actually exists a disease called "infertility" and that you may have contracted it?

You may be comfortable with this notion of infertility. It may even be part of your identity now. I want to encourage you to open yourself up to the idea that infertility does not have to apply to you. It does not have to be your identity.

In another chapter I'll be looking more closely at the potential damage the label and culture of "infertility" is promulgating in the Western world of medicine and pop culture today. But for right now, I'm suggesting that it's worthwhile to notice what you've decided about your own fertility, your identity, and what's trending in your mind related to it.

Above I mentioned that you are more than your fertility, because you are a whole person with a whole life. It is within your domain to live that whole life or not. Your fertility is reflected in many different areas of your life. "But how do I get the fertility in my womb to be what I want it to be?" you may be asking. You focus on it as fertile.

It can be scary to claim fertility for yourself after you've been disappointed by unfulfilled expectations. I'm inviting you to move back toward that claim with me. I know it's scary when you feel that you've failed and you're hurting. It may even feel like you're jinxing yourself if you boldly claim your fertility. But we are going to claim this for you so you can move forward toward motherhood, if that's what you want. If we stay in the identity of "infertility," how can we create? To create, we must be fertile.

Let's go slowly together and take some time to reflect on what "fertile" actually means. How do you define it? From the definition that you give it, reflect on your own life experience and see what you can find that reflects your fertility back to you. It might be useful to write it down. What have you created in your life?

A power move in the area of managing your mind around fertility is to control what feeds are coming to you. What news are you tracking about fertility? What Facebook groups and posts are you reading about fertility? What's the attitude and mindset of these groups or sources of information? If you are tracking, reading, or consuming anything that does not support the expansion of your fertility, I encourage you to omit it. What you focus on you find; what you focus on grows; what you focus on you become.

Be sure to fill the gap of what you omitted with fertile feeds. Find Facebook groups and news sources that focus on how women are enhancing their fertility and focusing on fertile ideas, the move into motherhood and babies, the active releasing of stories that don't serve fertility. Really anything that gets your happy, creative juices flowing can contribute to the enhancement of your fertility.

So Much Righteousness

The last unseen defeating residue that we'll examine here is the area of social judgment and righteousness. Again there is a lot of strong opinion and noise about what motherhood should be or what a person struggling to become a mother should do. Some of the noise comes to you from the inside. That's the source that's the most powerful.

The exercise here is to look at your notions about bringing new life into the world today. Once you've notice what you are thinking and feeling about it, decide what supports your fertility and what does not. What is serving you as you move toward becoming a mother and what is not?

Becoming a mother is really not about guilt or worthiness, although many of us can experience a conversation within ourselves that points to both of these. For example, I've already shared with you my own concerns regarding my standards for what a good mother looks like and how I could never live up to that.

For me, there was also the guilt factor in the mix. I've always been one to rescue companion animals. I just couldn't see not adopting an animal that already needed a home. So when I was stepping onto the path leading to parenthood, this "should" came up with a lot of guilt for me – I should adopt, right? Just like the kitties and puppies, there are already tons of kiddos who need a home; why make more?

Arguing the truth of these judgments is not what's useful. Rather, what's useful to share here is that part of my movement forward was making my claim as a neutral fact without guilt that my partner and I wanted to create our own baby. The truth here is that making our own baby was our hearts' desire. This is independent of anyone else's judgments. It was our own judgments that we had to modify to align with our hearts.

Part 4

Re-Membering

"The breeze at dawn has secrets to tell you.
Don't go back to sleep.
You must ask for what you really want.
Don't go back to sleep.
People are going back and forth across the doorsill
where the two worlds touch.
The door is round and open.
Don't go back to sleep."

– Rumi

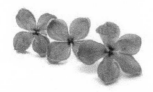

Chapter 8
Seeing Blood:
Grief and Healing

Whether we lose a baby through miscarriage, stillbirth, or termination, we experience grief. These causes of grief may seem very obvious. And then there's the less obvious – the grief that happens month after month of trying to conceive only to reluctantly experience the arrival of your monthly period. All of these instances of an abrupt end to a hopeful beginning are painful and leave their mark on us. In this section, we explore each of these scenarios not only for what is lost, but also for what is gained.

No matter which type of loss you are experiencing, allow yourself to accept that you've had loss, and allow yourself to grieve. There are many ways to do this. I'll conclude this chapter with some suggestions that apply to these types of loss. First let's explore monthly compounding loss, termination, miscarriage, and stillbirth separately.

Still Not Pregnant

Do you remember the first time you intentionally tried to get pregnant? The instant when you knew you were going to ovulate and made love in the right window of time and then tuned into every little twinge and tingle in your abdomen until the day your unwanted period showed up? For me this was before I even started the obsessive trap of peeing on sticks twice a month – once to detect ovulation, and then again to detect pregnancy.

I would be putting it mildly to say I was disappointed, and at the same time my confidence was low going in. I'm not sure why, but I was a doubter. Maybe it was because of those few times in high school that I had unprotected sex dangerously close to ovulation but thankfully didn't get pregnant. Whatever the reason, I was pessimistic.

And so, that first try felt like a confirmation of doom for me. But I am resilient. And so are you. That's why we keep trying even when we see blood month after month of diligently tracking, measuring, and planning our activities to maximize our fertility based on solid scientific information.

My favorite resource at that time was Toni Weschler's ever-popular *Taking Charge of Your Fertility*. You know the one, right? The well-known book can help you understand your cycle and get on the train to follow your body's measurable signals either to avoid or to achieve pregnancy. It's also a great resource for being your body's best care taker and advocate. Knowing what is happening with your cycle is very empowering and it helps to inform the conversations you're having with your healthcare providers.

Eventually for me, though, since I still wasn't getting pregnant, the exercise of tracking, measuring and then taking action in accordance with what was trending in my cycle started to feel like watching water boil. I wasn't getting any new information, and the information I had from my cycle was that I should be getting pregnant with ease. This was a first clue that there was more in the way of my parenthood than my biochemistry. I should have felt confident to know that my body was functioning right on par. I was sensing an inkling of this, but I couldn't see it clearly yet.

However, what I *could* see clearly was that it just wasn't happening for me. The more I focused on the fact that I wasn't getting the result I wanted, the more I got that disappointing result. If all signs pointed to my cycles being normal, what was wrong with my body? I've heard similar stories from other women, including some of my clients.

After many moons of this same disappointment, seeing the arrival of my period every month that I had tried to get pregnant literally made me cry. This was grief – the experience of loss. Every month I made a contract with my body to make a baby. Every month I felt that my body had failed.

In legal terms this is called expectation loss and is defined as a loss resulting from the inability to complete a contract by another's breach of the contract. Framing it this way, I could blame my body; but that only made me feel really crappy about myself and my body on top of the sadness of losing the expected baby that never was. It's an awful experience, and this grief is not really recognized or talked about.

There's a big difference in response from friends, family, and the medical establishment when you talk about trying to conceive and not achieving pregnancy versus when you talk about trying to conceive, getting pregnant, and then losing the pregnancy. I personally experienced the difference in response to the monthly loss, the early miscarriage loss, and the late-term loss. It's as if the zeitgeist has established a scale of difficulty and pain that ramps up depending on how far along the pregnancy is (or isn't).

While the pain is more obvious to others the longer the pregnancy has been medically recognized as a pregnancy, it is of course still very real and still hurts no matter when the loss occurs. For me, the level of shock and surprise increased as the time grew between trying to conceive and the expected delivery of a vibrant baby, but it all equates to pain, loss, and grief. Let's not fool ourselves.

So we're clear on what is lost; but what can we gain by the recurrence of our menstruation when we're looking for a pregnancy instead? There is opportunity in the fact that we *are* menstruating. The beautiful miracle that is our body is doing the monthly renewal process, preparing the womb for a future tenant – our baby. The fact that menstruation is happening means there is hormonal activity moving our reproductive potential through the cycle of egg prep and release, open season to receive sperm, preparation of the womb, and then refresh and renew when no pregnancy has taken place.

The length of the cycle is determined by the number of days from the first day of blood through the cycle to the next first day of blood (beginning of menses). How many days there are between each cycle gives us information about the hormonal functioning and the regularity of ovulation. So, we can celebrate that we have information to work with here that gives us clues about some of the physical elements of our game.

Before we move on to other sources of loss and grief in the pursuit of parenthood, I want to acknowledge that getting your period over and over again when what you're looking for is a pregnancy is painful. It is the experience of compounding grief. It's not a grief that's commonly acknowledged, and so it's not something we readily recognize. The tedious repetition of intention followed by action, followed by an unwanted result, hurts and accumulates.

Embracing the Loss in Termination

Termination of a pregnancy can deliver an unexpected complexity of emotions. Although in the case of termination there has been a reason that we choose to go the route of loss, the anguish can nonetheless go deep. It's common that this heartache is not given space, but grief following termination can be as intensely impactful as that of miscarriage or stillbirth. After having intentionally chosen abortion, grief can come as a surprise and therefore be unexpectedly overwhelming. Despite the choice to terminate, grief and guilt are real and common companions.

If you can relate to this type of loss, I know you had good reasons to choose abortion; I have not personally met anyone who takes it lightly. I can only imagine how difficult it is to come to this decision in the first place, and then to come to terms with the pain of this loss exacerbated by the guilt. It has been my privilege to witness this feat of courage and strength, and I honor you.

This was the case for Julianna, who had terminated three times before actively trying to become a mom. She chose to terminate the first two times because she recognized she was an alcoholic and, on top of that, she was not in a relationship nor in a position as a single mother to adequately support a newborn. I admire her wisdom and ability to respond to her situation in a way that would impact fewer lives. Her decision to terminate a third time was the sacrifice she made to stay in a stable relationship with a man who found parenthood non-negotiable.

Whatever someone's feelings might be about termination, each of us has to make our own choices and take actions to respond to the circumstances at hand in the best way we know how. All three of these terminations left their mark in Julianna's heart despite her belief that in each instance it was the best option at the time.

Fast forward to her readiness and desire to be a mom. Because of the previous pregnancies, she was sure that she would have no problem conceiving again. She was wrong. She wondered what was different now that she felt ready to receive the blessing of a baby. Through exploring her beliefs and deep feelings, she discovered that she was carrying heavy, heavy guilt and grief around her losses through termination. She struggled to reconcile her worthiness to be a mom now in light of the fact that she had passed up these previous opportunities.

Through creative grief processing and commitment to self-forgiveness and unconditional love, Julianna was able to embrace and then release the guilt and come to terms with the grief. This is hard work, clearing at a deep energetic level. She was able to tap into the places in her body where she was storing these wounds to process the releases. I admire her faith and dedication. Ultimately, Julianna chose to stay diligent with her commitment to Alcoholics Anonymous and focus her mothering instincts on rescue dogs.

Sometimes women who have struggled to achieve pregnancy also make the difficult decision to terminate. If you can relate to this experience, then you know first-hand that in these difficult cases, the reason is typically to avoid future suffering when abnormalities are found in the pregnancy through amniocentesis and ultrasound. There is profound loss here, and it includes immense physical and emotional stress.

When this happens, there is grief not only over the loss of the baby, but also over your lost dream of motherhood and lost faith in your body. It's critical to be with this grief rather than minimizing it and thinking that courage is getting over it and moving on. The courageous thing here is in accepting that this is real grief, that it takes time to process the feelings of the experience as well as the physical healing.

The First 10 Yards

Unfortunately, miscarriage is more common than we are led to believe. Sometimes we have the blessing of them going unnoticed, thank you. But other times, they deliver us pain no matter how big or little our growing baby is.

We are hit with a blow that interferes with the flow of our breath and our faith. There are so many unanswered questions and often no real way to get the information our brains need to make sense of it and know confidently how to prevent this experience from happening again. We feel caught in the in-between spot of having been an expectant mother for such a brief time before the high is sucked out of us, dashing us against the rocks. Can we really get back up and try this again?

Sometimes we know for sure because nurses and doctors get involved and we have confirmation that we miscarried. Other times we have no medical confirmation of pregnancy, but still we know, and the confirmation comes in the form of the nightmare of a very late, painful, and heavy period.

How can we prepare ourselves for the possibility of this misfortune? To do so seems in such opposition to the very outcome we are seeking. And although the creation of the lost conception was a team sport, the loss leaves us on the sidelines, holding the ball all alone.

We are strong. We cry. We grieve. We accept the truth. And we try again.

The Last 10 Yards

For me, stillbirth was not even on my radar. I thought I was home-free as I entered my third trimester. Boy, was I wrong.

In Chapter 1 – An Initiation by Fire into Peace I told the story of my journey to parenthood. It includes the soul-ripping stillbirth of my angel baby Ava Catherine. It was the bottom-of-the-barrel place I went to before there was no possible direction left but up. Nothing worse could happen to me after that. As broken as I felt, during my healing time I became indestructible. I had lived through what was for me unimaginable; it did not kill me.

There is a nightmare quality to knowing your baby has died and you are carrying her around until the time you deliver her. You will labor and deliver. It will hurt, emotionally and physically, like nothing you can dream up, but it will not kill you.

So is it better to not know until you've gone through the labor and delivery that your baby has died, or is it easier to know in advance? Either way, you have the starring role in your own nightmare.

Some of us will want to completely check out from this reality – the psyche is overloaded. Others will reach for distracting engagement, clinging to what and who is present with us. With either coping strategy we move ourselves away from being directly in the emotional pain. It's a weird twilight zone that's hard to describe.

Despite its tragic nature, there are gifts in this experience as well. The gifts that I received in this pregnancy include the validation that I was fully capable of conceiving and carrying a healthy baby (almost) to term; the experience of a flavor of love that I had previously never tasted; and the loving interaction between my mother and father that I did not remember seeing my entire life till we lost Ava. Those are just three of the gifts that I can identify. I encourage you to search your losses and make meaning of your experiences in a way that offers you gifts along with sorrows.

No matter how we come to experience our losses, they make a profound mark on our hearts and souls. In each of the scenarios of loss that we've explored here, there are multiple losses to grieve. There is the loss of the dream of motherhood and the loss of faith in the body we are relying on to bring us our cherished baby, and there is the loss of the baby.

The common thread in the healing process for each scenario is in the initial acceptance of loss and grief. Let it flow into you and out of you, over you and past you. Be in the waves; let them carry you. You will find that they will eventually carry you back to shore where you can slowly reestablish your footing. But understand that this takes patience and gentleness.

The wounds can go excruciatingly deep. There is rest and work to do. First rest. Rest into the acceptance process. Surrender yourself to the pain and the expression of the pain through tears and vocalizations, through writing and drawing. If you have the blessing of someone who can hold space for you while you experience the pain, allow them to be there for you, to listen and witness without fixing. Most likely you will need to hire this person to hold space for you – it's a rare skill and you need an experienced expert right now.

Then there is the work of accepting yourself and your body. And from acceptance you move through healing. Creative grief work enables a re-membering of yourself, your identity, and your heart after such harrowing splintering and shattering. The pieces can be gathered and reassembled. You are changed. And you come to a time for making meaning in a way that supports you to continue this life, and possibly your pursuit of parenthood. Arriving at the banks of the river of meaning takes a while following this kind of disintegration, but we all eventually get there. The way you make meaning will define the next version of you and how you move back into life.

An important piece in the process of making meaning is the realization or assignment, as the case may be, of the gifts to be celebrated in each of these experiences. This might strike you as a jarring idea at first, but there is something here for us. Each experience of loss and grief and recovery is an illustration of our insurmountable spirit.

Through my own journey, I am able to recognize amazing courage and strength in myself. Sometimes we need it reflected back to us and validated by another. For me, that validation came from my partner, who, not long after we lost Ava, told me I am the most courageous person he knows. Whether that's a measurable fact or not is irrelevant.

That he sees me this way is valuable to my healing and our relationship. I understand that I am a force of nature.

As I witness and facilitate the process through these experiences with my sisters who come to me in the struggle, I recognize the power each of us is endowed with. Choice is always ours. How we wield our choice is what creates the unfolding of our experience of life even through the pain.

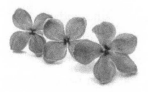

Chapter 9

Miracles: Can You Believe It?

I f choice is one of our superpowers, how do we know what our choices really are; how do we know what's possible? In this section we'll look at this question, and by the end you'll have a better sense of your bearings. The slippery, elusive part is that whatever is possible for you is something you already know. The challenge is in unearthing it so you can see it and move from there with confidence and courage. You are not as muddled as you might think.

How Do You Measure Up?

When you've been working at baby-making for a long time with disappointing results, it's helpful to understand your current biological and physical conditions clearly. So, if you haven't already, get the important hormones measured and understand your unique cycle.

Once you have a clear understanding of the biochemical and physical conditions, you will know what resources you need to bring things into more optimal working order. The guidance of a very trustworthy doctor or reproductive endocrinologist can be a boon in this discovery phase.

There are a few options to consider regarding how you want to approach balancing your hormones, if that's what's needed. As I mentioned in an earlier chapter, you can often attend to the hormones through nutritional therapy and emotional or stress management. These approaches are your best foundation for enhancing your fertility holistically as well as having a positive impact on your hormones. You may also want to get support from an acupuncturist, herbalist, or endocrinologist.

One thing that you can be sure of is that investing in an overall healthy lifestyle will deliver benefits in every area of your life well into the future. Adopting or adjusting healthy lifestyle practices now also sets you up to model good lifestyle choices as a parent. And as a pregnant mom, healthy lifestyle practices will support your pregnancy.

Know

We can get empirical information about our cycle and hormones from lab tests and the tracking that you can do at home each month. There are also other diagnostics that can be done with a doctor to make sure your fallopian tubes and ovaries are clear and that the shape and tilt of your womb are not creating an added level of complexity.

The other pieces of information are the ones we gather from within ourselves by observing our emotional states and triggers. What patterns of behavior have you been noticing since you've begun to move your attention toward your own thoughts and feelings? As you've noticed the direction of your thoughts, have you discovered anything that is lingering from your childhood that needs to be cleared? Do you need to spend some time diving in with your grief more deeply?

While the patterns of intertwined thoughts and emotions are sticky and often uncomfortable, these are the ones that will continue to pose obstacles for any physical treatments that you invest in. I believe that unwinding these inhibiting emotional patterns are where to focus your first investment. Find a reliable way to explore these areas before or in tandem with moving forward with physical treatments.

It's useful to have a method of talking with yourself that allows you to capture the conversation so you can reflect on what is said. Having someone guide these conversations can be helpful and make it a bit easier at first too. Some of my clients find journal dialoging works well when they are looking to reveal deeper truths.

You may also want to try using your breath to explore your body for information. Your body is constantly sending you information and messages about what it needs from you, the caretaker. As we discussed in an earlier section, it's important to be best allies with your body. Thank your body for all the good it has done for you today and all the good it will continue to do for you. Pledge that you will take good care of its needs. Not only will this carry you more smoothly down your path to parenthood, but it will also serve you for a long and vibrant life.

Be

When you have the information you need, you will understand the way that you are changing and shifting in response to the challenges you are facing. Every challenge brings us the opportunity to learn more deeply about ourselves and about the next best version of ourselves on the horizon.

Facing your fertility challenges is an opportunity to embody renewed possibility. You may experience the dawning of renewed possibility as you make your way through the aspects of self-exploration and life adjustment presented in Parts II and III of this book.

There is a new way of being on the horizon. You are becoming in every moment – becoming what you are growing into. If you are not pregnant but want to be, you are becoming pregnant. As your baby grows inside you, you are becoming a mother. As you learn to release the struggle and surrender to the process, you are becoming more at ease.

Do

Clarity, commitment, courage, and rigorous honesty with yourself will lead you to the right actions. When you confidently know the elements within your control, you are able to move forward. You are no longer muddled and conflicted, and therefore you are no longer overwhelmed and stuck.

Trying to move forward without clarity, commitment, courage, and rigorous honesty is like a hamster running in a wheel. You will expend a lot of effort, remain frustrated, and get nowhere. This type of activity comes at a great expense to your self-esteem, your energy, your bank account, and your relationships.

Here are a few items to keep on your To Do list for all time. Keep accepting where you are. Keep forgiving yourself any harm you have done to yourself. Keep choosing the way you want to respond instead of reacting the way you have automatically in the past. Keep taking small steps into the new version of you as you make those behavior choices in each moment. Over and over again you get to choose – the same or something different.

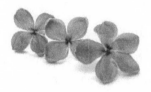

Chapter 10
Shift the Mind First: The Body Will Follow

Hold in your mind only what you want to create. Use "no" powerfully and use "yes" powerfully. The powerful "no" and the powerful "yes" both come from that state of clarity, commitment, courage, and rigorous honesty with yourself. Say no to the things (thoughts, feelings, activities) that do not serve and do not enhance your fertility. Say yes to the things (thoughts, feelings, activities) that do serve and enhance your fertility.

Fall in love with the process and the new possibilities. Through your decision to pursue parenthood, you have chosen to move toward a new you. You can never go back and you will never be the you that you were before. Celebrate the birthing of the new you as you journey on in a different frame of mind.

The More Fertile Mindset

Disciplining your imagination and focus is a powerful practice. We started out looking at the details of what's brought you to the life experiences you are now having, with the current highlight being challenges with fertility. That exercise is like putting all the puzzle pieces on the table, sorting out the edge pieces from the center pieces, and grouping pieces with similar colors together.

Then we looked at the vision and the picture you see for your life moving forward. This vision reveals potentials and possibilities. To be clear, it does not show you the how – it just shows you the what. After we have a clear understanding of the vision, we can know if the puzzle pieces we have in hand are the right ones to actually achieve that vision or not. If the picture in the pieces does not match the vision you are holding, you know it's time to break old patterns and habits and create new ones.

The process of breaking old patterns and developing new ones is an incremental process of reconditioning that happens little by little with your new awareness. You know you have a different choice; you know that in the moment an old pattern comes to the game, you can interrupt it and choose to play the new pattern – over and over again. By disciplining your imagination, you manage your focus and implement the reconditioning that roots in the new habits or patterns. This reconditioning solidifies the new patterns moving you toward what you are becoming. New established patterns are your new pieces that come together as your vision in order to achieve the outcome of your heart's desire.

Wear Your Best Pair of Glasses

Your focus defines your perspective, how you see things. Notice how you are already beginning to see things differently with the small shifts in perspective that you're experiencing as you read this book. What you focus on, you find. What you focus on grows. What you focus on seems real. And ultimately, what you focus on, you become.

Do you want to be as fertile as you can possibly be? Yes, you do. Then I ask you, what are you focusing on? Does that need to change?

You can manage your perspective and therefore your thoughts and feelings by disciplining your imagination and choosing what you are focusing on. This is so powerful it's almost magical. When you feel good, wonderful neurochemicals flow through your brain, triggering good chemical activity in your body and consequently better physical functionality. It's like a chain of dominoes. Your mind decides how the dominoes will tip and therefore how you see and experience life.

Draw the Line

How do you develop this sense of focus so you can channel your energy for your clarity, commitment, and courage? Decide what is not negotiable for you and set firm boundaries. Your boundaries are the lines that you draw based on your standards and values. This means to clearly say "no" about certain things and "yes" about others. There is no need to prove or justify the values and standards you are choosing.

Your boundaries will fortify you with the clarity, commitment, and courage that you have about the pursuit of your vision of parenthood and what's possible for you. You will experience renewed energy and strength from your inside out with your boundaries. And it is with your boundaries that you guide others in how they can treat you and what they can expect from you. This is great practice for parenting. Your child will benefit from your modeling good boundaries.

Movement

Life is dynamic, constantly changing and growing. There is no static moment. You can sit still, but you are still a dynamic being. Your breath, your blood, your cells, your thoughts and feelings are constantly in motion. You are built to move. Two years from today, every cell in your body will be different from the cells now present.

Follow your need to move and change. One of the simplest things your body requires from you is movement. Find ways to fulfill this need every day. It doesn't have to be a big deal. You don't need to run out and get a gym membership. You can simply do more walking. You can take stretch breaks. You can have spontaneous dance parties in your living room. You can join a yoga class. There are many, many easily accessible ways to incorporate movement into your daily life.

Put some of your focus on thinking of yourself as a mover. Become a mover. The practice of making and taking opportunities to move will feed into that enhancement of your fertility. To be clear, this is not about a specific exercise routine. Rather, like the disciplined imagination for managing the focus of your thoughts and feelings, the movement invokes the feel-good chemistry in the body. This is often underrated, and it's so very powerful.

Part 5

BIG BANG

"Any perception can connect us to reality properly and fully. What we see doesn't have to be pretty, particularly; we can appreciate anything that exists. There is some principle of magic in everything, some living quality. Something living, something real, is taking place in everything."

– excerpt from *The Sacred Path of the Warrior*, by Chögyam Trungpa

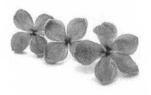

Chapter 11
Steps: Elements of Shift

Has your fertility journey overwhelmed you or brought you deep fatigue, extreme sadness, even a sense of helplessness? Roller coaster rides can be engaging and exciting at first, but if you stay on for too many cycles around the track, you eventually feel beaten, tossed around, and exhausted. You might be screaming to get off the ride while at the same time feeling driven to stay the course.

No matter how desperate you feel your situation is at this moment or how loud the tick of that biological clock, it's time to get off the ride, take a deep breath, lift your head up from the struggle, and reorient yourself to a more stable and even pace. Your body, your heart, and your relationships will all benefit from some relief.

A nurtured body is better able to do the work of conceiving and carrying a baby. As you experience relief, you can return to your relationship with your partner from a more open and loving space. You will see your choices and possibilities more clearly, more confidently, and more peacefully.

In this chapter, I present some simple and powerful steps you can gently take with yourself. In the following chapter, you'll find a set of new perspectives, or lenses, that support each step. Reviewing these steps and lenses frequently is the best way to receive the biggest benefit from them. Add journaling and you get what I like to call the "Big Bang" effect. Each time you internalize these concepts, perspectives, and steps, something new and deeper will evolve in you, taking you through a gradual and significant shift.

Step 1: Reconnect

Failing to conceive or losing a pregnancy can lead to feelings of anger and shame, which can then lead to isolation, loneliness, and marginality. Making it worse is the frustration that comes from having relatives and friends asking, "So when are you going to have kids?" Sometimes, they're a bit kinder and rephrase the question as something like, "Do you think you want kids some day?"

Either way, the question lands like a knife in your gut. The emotional weight of it is too huge, and even if you wanted to talk about it, they probably wouldn't understand.

What if you could leave that question behind? What if you could be free from trying for a minute? How would that feel? Close your eyes, take a deep breath, and imagine that.

Are you missing your friends? Are you missing the connection you had with them, the easy laughter and silly fun? Where has your lightness gone? It's in the trash with all those negative pregnancy tests.

We need our people, especially at a time like this. Despite our inclination to pull away, obsess, and hold our breath alone, our frustration and shame are soul cries for those easier times with the people who love you. It's time to get reconnected.

Your time and energy are sacred, therefore you must be extremely discerning about who you spend them with. Because you need to give and receive love from a variety of friends and family, you must do your part to nurture important relationships so they can in turn nurture you.

How does it feel to look at your relationships like this? What do you see? Who can be present with you? Who can you be present with?

Remember a time, maybe it was during college, or maybe it was a few years ago, when you spent time having fun with friends. Who did you love hanging out with? When was the last time you hung out with that person? What is it about this person that makes them special to you?

Being in a group may feel a bit overwhelming if you've been huddling under the "leave me alone, I'm feeling miserable" blanket for a while now. So think of just one or two friends or family members that you miss being with, who you can rely on to lift you up and share a laugh with. Decide to call or write to them. Let them know you'd like to talk or hang out and that you miss them.

As you reconnect, lay the ground rules right away. If you want to talk about your fertility challenges, for example, be sure to let your friend know you need her to listen without giving you suggestions or looking for a solution. You just want her to hear you. And if there are topics or conversations that are too difficult, let your friend know that these are areas that are too tender for you right now. Your friends and family who love you really do want to know how best to be there for you. They can only know if you tell them. Be gentle with them and yourself.

Communicate the rules of whatever you specifically do want or specifically don't want in this connection. Set your boundaries in a clear and gentle way that lets the other person know where you are and what you are available for.

Be honest. Own your experience and your feelings. Make no one else responsible for them. Let others be honest about theirs. And let them be responsible for theirs. This is the structure for healthy and ultimately mutually supportive relationships.

Each of us is doing the best we can within the realm of our experience. Friends and family members may be struggling with how to be with you, just as you are struggling with how to be with them. This exercise of connecting, setting boundaries, and honestly owning our feelings can be a hard one if it's new.

Remember, you are in control of your experience. You are the decision maker, the choice taker. Recognize and claim the truth of your thoughts and feelings. Acknowledge and allow for your true feelings and needs. Stay connected to important relationships by communicating and owning your experience and needs.

Step 2: Show Yourself the Love

Each cycle that unfolds on your fertility journey involves so much body attention, possibly more than you've ever focused in this way before. And it's completely different from the kinds of attention you might have given your body in the past.

Are you a person who actually prefers not to focus on your body at all? Has the attention you've put there while trying to conceive made you uncomfortable? Perhaps you used to enjoy working out, having sex, and other physical activities, but now you're just feeling so let down by your body that physical activity has lost its attraction.

Regarding conception, you've probably heard that it matters if you're underweight and it matters if you're overweight... and what weight is exactly perfect for conception anyway? That's enough to make us crazy right there. "Maybe if I hadn't eaten all those Pop-Tarts in college, or maybe if I.... Can I just get a new body already?" That was some of my self-talk when getting to motherhood wasn't working out like I had planned.

When you get to the body-hating part of the fertility journey, it's really time to take a *big,* deep breath and open the opportunity to reset the game board. Have a seat; have a cry; and then take a good loving look at your body.

Your body is sacred and valuable, therefore you must be a discerning caretaker and nurturer of it. Because your body enables all of your physical activities, you understand its great value to you and the variety of opportunities it has afforded you throughout all the phases of your life.

How does it feel to see your body this way? Can you remember some of the highlights that you've experienced in this body? Here are a few common activities that you may have taken for granted: swimming, walking, sexuality. Perhaps you've also enjoyed some less common physical opportunities; for example, horseback riding, playing an instrument, tight rope walking.... Well, you get my point. Your body has been there for you in so many ways all the days of your life.

Body appreciation is a hard pill to swallow for a lot of us on any given day. But when you feel completely let down by your body after unsuccessfully trying to be a mommy for so long, it seems nearly impossible. I'm inviting you to come to a place of loving relationship with your body.

Can you remember the time you felt the sun on your back and the wind in your hair? Did you recently take a refreshing shower? How wonderful does it feel to get your hair washed? And what about that delicious meal you were able to enjoy because of all those happy little taste buds on your tongue? These are all physical activities that we need a body for. Your body really is a magnificent thing.

If you haven't already conjured up happy-body memories, take a few moments now to do that. It's most powerful to actually write them down. Revisit all the phases and stages of life you've experienced so far, and identify physical experiences that put a smile on your face.

When you're in a place of feeling a bit softer toward your body and more appreciative of what it's already contributed to your life, let's go a little deeper. Consider what you've been demanding of your body lately. You've been asking it to deliver you a miracle, literally.

Did you know that over half of all pregnancies end in miscarriage? Many of them are early enough to be undetected, but of course, that's not always the case. The fact that any of us exists is truly a result of a very specific and precise moment in time when a whole recipe of ingredients came together just so.

Let your understanding of the detailed requirements for creating life give you a little space to take some pressure off. You are a human being with a human body dancing in a sea of possibilities. Your natural existence is the complete opposite of a controlled laboratory. Consider taking a break from treating your body like a lab and expecting yourself to perform like a precision chemist.

If we attack someone, it's natural that they retaliate, bracing themselves against us in defense. By contrast, if we approach someone with compassion and gentleness, inviting them to collaborate, they are more likely to trust and be open to us. On our fertility journey, we need our body's openness and cooperation. Send your body messages of compassion and love.

Each time you menstruate, your body is doing its house cleaning, preparing for the possibility of a future visitor. Some visitors are able to stay and some are not. Eventually, *all* visitors leave. Can you move into a feeling of supporting that process? Can you understand that your body is doing the best that it can with the resources that it has?

I know I'm asking a lot of you, especially if you've already been trying to do all the right things to prepare your body to conceive and carry. I know this particular step is long and steep. I know there is a massive weight on your back as you take this step of loving your body. I also know that you can do it.

I encourage you to be courageous; establish and maintain an appreciation and respect for all that your body has done and is doing on your behalf. Antagonism creates disconnect in any relationship.

To bolster your body appreciation and to create the essential ease in your relationship with your body, identify practices and activities that are uniquely enjoyable and supportive to your body. And then do them.

You are the decision maker, the choice taker. Choose gentleness and love for your body. You need your body and your body needs your care. Make this a healthy relationship, and then as you brush your teeth each night, smile big with gratitude for all the amazing adventures you're having in this body.

Step 3: Tame and Train the To Do List

The last step may have been a stretch and an invitation into uncomfortable territory, so in this step we'll keep it pragmatic with a look at time management. Getting the daily dragon of the To Do List under control is an easy way to achieve a sense of freedom and fresh air. Even if some of this is old news, stick with me. Consider if and how you are actually making your To Do List work for you at this critical time.

Depending on where you are on your fertility journey, you will have a variety of fertility-related items on the list. This added layer of demands on top of your career, relationships, and important weekly life tasks – like doing your laundry and getting some exercise – can make it a little hard to breathe. Your time, energy, and emotions are getting taxed to the max. The way you employ your To Do List can make a big difference in how you experience life each day.

Let's have a look at that long, heavy, hungry, ever-expanding To Do List (TDL) of yours. The TDL can be either a useful and happy employee or one of your most disgruntled workers.

The simple solution is to keep it useful. Let it process items of *highest value and highest priority* for you. It should collect and then push those items on, allowing for a freer mind and a sense of progress. Demand that the TDL work for you as a tunnel through which high priorities constantly flow. Maintain the flow.

Like all hard workers with high-demand bosses, a hard-working TDL needs an assistant – the calendar. Move high priorities from the TDL to a scheduled slot on the calendar. Let the calendar be a guide to keep the focus on those most valuable and important activities for the day. Always build in a buffer between scheduled activities and appointments, and always over-estimate how long something will take rather than cutting yourself short and creating a bungle of emotion and effort.

Do I hear you saying that you're already using your calendar in conjunction with your TDL *and* you're still feeling bullied, harried, and stressed? This situation leads to fatigue, frustration, and more stress. There are chemical, biological, and psychological consequences here. Let's make that TDL earn its keep.

Your time and energy are sacred, therefore you must be extremely discerning about where you spend them.

How does your TDL look from that angle? Do you see things on your list that are definitely *not* high priorities?

Are you using a Low Priority List yet? The Low Priority List also holds things you want to do, but it's specifically for things that are not high priorities. What is on your current TDL that does not qualify as high value and high priority? Move those to your Low Priority List now.

Next, ask yourself, "What would the consequence be if I let this item go and dropped it from my list completely?"

While you focus on the high priorities, see if you can get more and more comfortable with letting go of some of the low priority items. I usually find that a handful of low priority items are of no consequence.

You'll recognize these items by the way they stay on your list for a long time doing nothing more than creating stress. Often, I conclude that these items have no real value to me or I would have gotten to them already. If they are actually high-value items that you just don't have the bandwidth for, can they be delegated?

Sometimes we take on tasks that actually belong to someone else. I want to remind you to recognize that it's perfectly appropriate to tell whoever actually owns those To Do items that you cannot be responsible for them right now. You do not have space for it right now.

When we return the responsibility to its owner, we create an opportunity for that person to make an informed decision about the task, and we've responsibly admitted that we are not available for it right now. If drama comes up for the person in reaction to your communication, be a witness, not a participant – and then leave it there. You have high priorities of your own calling your attention.

By the way, letting responsibility be held by its rightful owner is an advanced skill for successful mothering. It acknowledges the other person's capability and enables their independence. Take the opportunity to practice now.

Every time you have something you want to add to your TDL, declare out loud, "My time and energy are sacred, therefore I am extremely discerning about where I spend them." Revisit and reevaluate your Low Priority List from time to time. If you find that there are items there that have gained value or priority for you, assign them to your calendar. The ultimate resting place for each To Do is in a scheduled time slot where it will actually be addressed. Maintain the flow.

You are the decision maker, the choice taker. Master these powers by applying the process of carefully considering items that want to jump onto your precious TDL and putting them in their appropriate place. Be a discerning gatekeeper of your time and energy.

Step 4: Meet the Dancing Heart

When we are wanting a baby and it is unexpectedly difficult, we long to escape from the diminishing hope, growing anger, and mounting frustration. The darkness grows with the passing of each cycle. We sense that our feelings are not supportive to conceiving and carrying to term. We recognize that we must do something effective and powerful to change the course of the journey.

I want to guide you back to your heart. It's the sacred space from which all our creations are sourced and from which all our wisdom flows. Because your heart reveals to you everything you need to know, feel, and see, I encourage you to tune in and open up in a deep and clearing way on a regular basis. Entering the sacred heart space provides a unique process that supports your peace and ease.

Give yourself time and space for this one. Make arrangements to be completely alone. Make an appointment with yourself and honor it in the same way you would an appointment with your doctor. This remedy is important and powerful medicine. Deeply take in that knowing and the expectation. With this process we are creating a meeting space for you and your relief.

Still and quiet are best achieved when you can be completely alone. Alone includes turning off or unplugging all electronic devices. And when you try a practice of still and quiet for the first time, I recommend no music. Nothing but the sounds, smells, and surrounding elements that are generally unchangeable or out of your control.

Once you've arranged your time and space and you've created a supportive environment, sit in a comfortable position where your bottom and your back are softly but firmly supported. Find a chair that is soft and wide or a couch you can sink into. Sit so your feet are supported flat on the floor and your arms can hang in a relaxed way with your hands separately resting in your lap. Hold your head upright with a relaxed neck. Close your eyes.

Take a deep, cleansing breath... and another... and another. On each exhalation, let go of the places in your body where you are holding things together, where your muscles are contracted. Think soft, squishy, loose, limp. Continue to enjoy deep, cleansing breaths. Allow your body to rest gently back into the support behind you. Melt a little... melt a little more. Breathe.

With your eyes still closed and your breath flowing in and out slowly and deeply, move your awareness to the center of your chest where your heart is. Imagine a big heart shape right there in the center of your body – three dimensions taking up space from front to back and from below your neck to just above your belly. Give the heart a color that feels good to you; fill it with gold or pink or purple or green – whatever color brings you a sense of lightness and happiness as you picture it.

Now give your heart movement; imagine your beautiful, colorful heart in a synchronized dance with your breath. As your breath flows in, your magnificent heart moves – perhaps it sparkles or radiates or expands. As your breath flows out, your magnificent heart continues to move –perhaps it glows a different color or bows or turns. Continue your heart dance with your breath – your breath is the rhythm, and your colorful heart is the dancer. Sit and watch. Breathe and enjoy the rhythm and the movement.

Fully experience the brilliance, love, freedom, warmth, and glow of your Dancing Heart in the quiet stillness here. The only movement is the cadence of your breath and your colorful heart.

As your heart continues the dance, move your awareness to its very center. Here at the center of your beautiful, colorful Dancing Heart, the wonderful people and things that are in your life are revealed to you in a way that shows you their value and reminds you of the reasons you love them. As you focus on the Dancing Heart, ask yourself who or what is in my life that brings me joy, makes me laugh, gives me that special feeling I enjoy?

Perhaps you see the place you live and how it keeps you safe and warm. Perhaps you see your pets and how they give you affection and are happy to see you no matter what. Perhaps you see a favorite piece of clothing that makes you feel particularly comfortable. You might even see yourself and recognize how very courageous you are. The possibilities are endless.

It's likely that you'll notice some things you have taken for granted or have forgotten. It's a delight to remember them. Feel the love that rises here. Drink it in. Savor it. This love is in you – always.

When you are ready to end the process and prepare to move back into the day that you left behind for this sacred interlude, be gentle with yourself. If your eyes are open and you're no longer focusing on your breath, go back to the space of quiet and still with closed eyes and slow, deep, cleansing breaths.

When you are feeling full of this light and love and rhythm of the Dancing Heart, bring your awareness back to your whole body. Imagine waving a farewell to your colorful Dancing Heart – perhaps blow it a kiss. Scrunch and wiggle your toes, stretch your legs. Open your eyes, stretch your arms.

And now gently smile. No matter what thoughts or feelings you are having right now, smile; keep breathing while you hold the smile for a moment. When you feel ready, get up and reenter the day.

This process of being with the Dancing Heart may create an emotional break-up for you. You may cry or laugh, or possibly both simultaneously. All of these possibilities are perfect. Go with the emotions. Let them flow. Give yourself this opening to express and relieve some of your pressure.

Those tight, brittle nuggets that you've been compacting way deep in your soul are being dissolved and given the opportunity to reintegrate in a way that is more supportive to you. Let it happen. Look forward to it. This cleansing can bring you rejuvenation and the energy you need to continue on your path to parenthood. You may not notice much progress at first, but if you commit to the practice and keep your meetings with your Dancing Heart, you will experience the benefit.

The emotional break-up may feel confusing because of the variety of emotions released and experienced in such a powerful way. Know that you are safe. Know that you are still whole. Know that enabling this experience creates new opportunities and possibilities for you.

What did you learn from your Dancing Heart? Did you receive important reminders about people and things that are good in your life? Are there things you forgot about that you like to do? How can you bring some of that back into your life right now?

This Dancing Heart space is with you wherever you are. All you need to create is the quiet stillness to enable the process. Go there when you need to. Go there on a regular basis so that the need is met even when you forget or want to ignore the need. These appointments don't have to be long. Create the time/space that fits into your life and keep your Dancing Heart appointments.

You are in control of your experience. You are the decision maker, the choice taker. The Dancing Heart process is important and powerful medicine for your aching soul. Write your own prescription, and administer your own dosage. As you continue your fertility journey, you can enjoy a sense of renewed spaciousness and hope on a path that can sometimes feel like a field of land mines. Stay connected to the wisdom and power of your heart.

I've made an audio recording of The Dancing Heart Guided Meditation for you. It's a resource to use as a practice over and over again. I hope you'll find it to be a refuge as you cross the stormy sea. It's one of my gifts to you in the Fertile Foundations Toolkit.

Step 5: Do the Quality Quench

Mmmmm... drinking cool water delivers an instant uplift and relieves that heavy feeling of fatigue. Now I know you've been told about hydration before, but please hang with me as we deepen our understanding of why water is vital on the path to relief as you struggle with fertility challenges. The cool temperature of the water in your mouth and on your throat will temporarily draw blood up to your head, giving you a natural shot of energy. Ahhh... feel the fog clear, and then keep drinking for more cool relief.

The simple action of drinking more water every day makes a world of difference to our energy level, complexion, and our digestion too. In fact, all the systems of the body benefit, including the reproductive system. Water is the fundamental building block for every human cell. Establish this healthy habit now so that your body and your baby's growing body will be sufficiently watered.

The Mayo Clinic has a wonderful diagram that illustrates many ways that water supports the body and its systems. If you're curious, check out "Functions of Water in the Body" from the Mayo Clinic. You can clearly see that nearly all of the major systems in your body depend on water.

Your body and your energy are sacred, therefore you drink to energize yourself and to hydrate and support your body's systems and functions by choosing quality quenchers. Your intention to maintain sufficient hydration is easy to accomplish because you plan for and have easily accessible healthy drinks on hand.

How does the idea of staying better hydrated throughout each day feel when you consider your intention this way? Do you have good reasons to incorporate conscious choice around what, how, and how often you'll drink? After a week or two of including a hydration plan in your life, you'll feel the improvement.

You are the decision maker, the choice taker. Master your drink domain and reap the benefits of vibrancy, clarity, and health. Be a discerning gatekeeper of your body and energy. As you continue your fertility journey, you can feel the uplifting and energizing effect of good hydration. If you've been used to living with dehydration, you may find relief from headaches, lightheadedness, dizzy spells, back aches, joint aches, fatigue, and menstrual cycle irregularities.

Step 6: Fortify Your Foundation

It's my intention that you find these steps alone are a good start for getting relief from the challenges you are facing right now. You may also realize that you need more specific support working through a process, or that you'd like to go deeper and bring in support that can reach even further into the weekly ups and downs of your fertility journey. These steps have worked well for me and for my coaching clients, and I know they can serve you.

Here's a final exercise for this chapter on shift. Close your eyes and imagine the feeling of limitless possibility, like a wide open field of tall grass moving in a gentle wind. Imagine yourself in the middle of this field of possibility. Feel yourself opening to the possibility that your journey can be easier. When you feel open, ask yourself:

- What is it that I want?
- What qualities of experience do I want to have?
- What feelings and experiences am I pursuing?
- How can I create those desired feelings and experiences within myself and my life?
- What are the choices I have made recently that are creating the experience I am having now?
- Which of those choices am I now willing to change, so that I can change the experience I am having?
- Who can support me in the process of recognizing my choices?
- Who can support me in the process of making new choices?

- Who can I consistently rely on to be there for me as I embody my new way of being and create my desired experience?
- Who can understand the experience I'm having and help me move toward my desired experience?

Are you getting answers to the questions above? Sometimes the answers pop right up. Sometimes they need a little coaxing out. If you are not getting the answers right away, or if the answers seem vague and foggy, or if the questions themselves are not quite making sense, give yourself some time with them. Let them wash over you and settle in. Read them over, put them aside, come back to them later, and see what arises. You may want to do this process more than once.

When we are faced with difficulties and we continue to struggle with the challenges alone, we eventually run out of ways to see the problem. Our perspective becomes stuck and stagnant. There is no progress; there is only frustration. While it would have been nice to have a sturdy, insightful helper from the beginning, there comes a time when we know we can no longer continue without help.

Is there a trusted friend you can reach out to? Even better, is there someone you trust to love and support you who has previously gone through what you're experiencing now? See if she can be there for you. People cannot help you if you don't let them know you need it. And then open yourself to receive that support.

If you have been relying on friends and family for their love and support and that's *not* providing the solution and comfort you were hoping for, or if you are not certain about sharing your burden with them, or if you simply don't have that option, look outside of your usual circle. Find a group or a trusted authority that is able to be there for you in the way that you need.

You are in control of your experience. You are the decision maker, the choice taker. The frustration you are feeling right now about your fertility challenges and your experience on the path to parenthood may be creating an overwhelming life of deep fatigue. The roller coaster ride you're on will eventually – if it hasn't already – leave you and your relationships with deep bruises.

You don't have to give up your dreams, but you do want to look at how you are experiencing the manifestation of those dreams. You are truly not alone and every step on the path can be taken from a place of either struggle or ease.

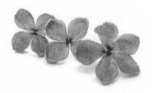

Chapter 12

Lenses: New Point of View

I n this chapter, I've collected the new points of view presented in the six steps of the previous chapter to help you shift your perspective. Think of them as new lenses through which to see your situation and your choices within the situation. These lenses are the positive statements that you can use to change the way you think and therefore feel, leading you to feel infinitely better, less hopeless, and more empowered.

Use these statements not only as a way to look at the situation differently in the moment, but also as affirmations and reminders. Affirming them to yourself regularly will recondition your mind and what you are focusing on. This practice works in your favor to keep your perspective healthy and supportive. Many of my clients find it helpful to use a journal and take notes about how and where specifically you want to apply these perspectives in your life.

You'll notice that some of these are longer than most affirmations. This is another reason to focus on them one at a time. They are intentionally written in fullness to deliver a specific vibrational effect. They also require more attention and effort to memorize. They can command your focus and powerfully shift your perspective if you let them.

Ways to Embody the New Lenses

One of the best ways to embody new perspectives or affirmations is to choose one at a time to focus on for a couple of weeks. Write it out once a day in a dedicated journal. Use the journal to note what you are experiencing in relation to the new perspective – how it's working for you and the situations in which you are applying it during your day. Focus on one at a time until it's truly part of you.

Another powerful way to anchor new perspectives is to record yourself saying them. Play them back to yourself in your own voice daily or even multiple times a day for a few weeks. Again you may want to focus on one at a time.

Big Bang

Doing both practices together of journaling and listening to an audio recording delivers a most powerful punch. As you begin to know them by heart, stand in front of a mirror, look yourself in the eyes, and say the affirming statement out loud. As you get more comfortable with saying it to yourself in the mirror, add emotion to the words; feel them as you say them, giving them more effect. Feel them in your body. Smile at yourself with love!

Lens 1: Relationships

My time and energy are sacred, therefore I am extremely discerning about who I spend them with.

Because I need to give and receive love from a variety of friends and family, I do my part to nurture important relationships.

Lens 2: Self-Acceptance, Self-Love, and Self-Nurturance

My body is sacred and valuable, therefore I am a discerning caretaker and nurturer of my body.

Because my body enables all of my physical activities, I understand its great value to me and the variety of opportunities it has afforded me throughout all the phases of my life.

Lens 3: Time and Energy

My time and energy are sacred, therefore I am extremely discerning about where I spend them.

Lens 4: Sacred Heart

My heart is the sacred space from which all my creations are sourced and from which all my wisdom flows.

Because my heart reveals to me everything I need to know, feel, and see, I commit to tuning in and opening up in a deep way on a regular basis.

I understand that entering the sacred heart space provides me with the unique healing process that is essential to my peace and ease.

Lens 5: *Essential Hydration*

My body and my energy are sacred, therefore I drink to energize myself and to hydrate and support my body's systems and functions by choosing quality hydration.

My intention to maintain sufficient hydration is easy to accomplish, because I plan for and have easily accessible healthy drinks on hand.

Lens 6: *My Choice*

My life can be as joyful as I want it to be. I choose to experience ease and peace no matter what appears on my path.

Because my life is sacred, I am aware of the choices that are mine to make and discerning about how I am experiencing in my life.

My choices create an experience free of struggle and conflict.

Part 6

In the End

"When you focus on your vision and discipline your imagination, you become a mega-star. You're not just successful, you're outrageously successful. We all have access to future possibility through our imagination. Memory does not create. Only imagination creates. Imagination. Use it to create the future you want for yourself."

– excerpt from *Are You Up For the Challenge?*,
by Rod Hairston

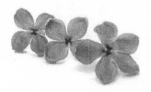

Chapter 13
From the Trenches

I t's my sincere hope that as you read this book, you experience a shift toward ease in your struggle with your fertility. One thing I know for certain is that shifting from struggle to ease on your journey to parenthood is a wonderful investment in your fertility and overall well-being.

It's one thing to read about something, it's another thing to implement and embody new perspectives and habits. Every client has unique aspects to their particular journey and story when I meet them, but one commonality is the neglect of self-nurturing and self-care and a tendency toward perfectionism and control. These trends make it even more difficult to make your way toward ease. It takes time and patience and dedicated, repetitive practice. You can do this on your own or you can recruit help. I know of at least ten benefits of working with someone's support in moving toward something you want that feels out of reach. Your support person or coach:

1. Provides a structure of accountability, which frees you up to know you're going to make progress through actions you and your coach agree upon
2. Consistently holds your belief for you while you grow into it
3. Consistently practices compassion, acceptance, and empathy toward you
4. Consistently holds up a model of what you are becoming with your new thoughts, feelings, and behavior patterns
5. Acts as a reliable cheerleader who is always on your team
6. Challenges you to make what seems impossible possible by partnering with you to creatively find solutions
7. Consistently keeps your vision a priority so that you yourself can practice keeping it a priority
8. Recognizes and celebrates every milestone you make no matter how small
9. Provides reliable companionship on the journey so you are not alone
10. Increases your probability of a successful shift by 95%

I've seen these benefits with my own clients, experienced them in my own life, and I've read many studies that have come to the same conclusions.

There are ten parallel obstacles that come up when we try doing it alone.

1. Can you create a structure of accountability? If not, it often results in a preoccupation with whether you are going to

succeed or fail to make progress distracting you from actually making progress.

2. Can you consistently hold your new belief for yourself while you are growing into it? This is an extra layer of challenge and demands powerfully disciplined imagination.

3. Can you consistently practice compassion, acceptance, and empathy toward yourself? You can check into this by noticing what your self-talk sounds like today.

4. Can you consistently hold and model an image of what you are becoming with your new thoughts, feelings, and behavior patterns?

5. Can you be your own most reliable cheerleader who is always on your team?

6. Can you challenge yourself to make what seems impossible possible by creatively finding solutions on your own?

7. Can you consistently keep your vision of what you are becoming and the life you are moving toward a priority so that it can become a reality?

8. Can you recognize and celebrate every milestone you make no matter how small? And how does it feel when you do this alone compared to sharing these milestones with a trusted companion?

9. Do you have at least one companion on this journey who is not occupied with their own struggles?

10. What's the probability of a successful shift if you are doing it without support?

Fundamentally Difficult

Let's not pretend. It's hard to release struggle. We've grown attached to the struggle to the degree that it is currently part of our identity, part of the way we see ourselves living life right now. It's hard to see different possibilities. We've been disappointed and emotionally broken down repeatedly by now, and mustering the energy without an outside spark is daunting to say the least. It's hard to create ease on your own without the help of outside resources and reinforcement because your internal resources are tapped out. If they weren't, you probably wouldn't be reading this book.

If you'd like to explore what it could be like to move through your journey to parenthood with more peace in your heart and ease in your life, please join me in a complimentary clarity session. During your session, I will help you get crystal clear about how you can stop struggling and move forward from a place of confident choice again. Most people begin to feel better during the first 15 minutes. It's one of my presents to you in the Fertile Foundations Toolkit.

I'll end this chapter with one of my favorite stories from the fertility journey of one of my coaching clients. Let it inspire you and kindle warmth for your soul and light for your psyche, assuring you that there is a way out of the darkness. Everyone's path is different, but there is a common message of renewed possibility here.

The Impossibility of Natural Conception

When Cathy came to me, she was in her mid-30s and dedicated to her work with special needs students. Despite trying for almost two years, she and her spouse had not been able to conceive. She was frustrated with the responses that she was getting from her doctors, who were focused on taking an aggressive approach to her fertility. They felt that she was experiencing compromised fertility because of endometriosis. Cathy also had been treating a thyroid condition and inflammation with medication for a number of years. She was committed to her work and the needs of family members who required extra support for different reasons. Her diet was defined by convenience and comfort, and she often had trouble falling asleep at night.

Her main complaints and challenges as she described them to me were feeling overwhelmed about having so many decisions to make moving through her fertility journey and feeling like she was doing it alone. She also wanted someone to help her deal with all the ups and downs that she was experiencing. She wanted support so that she wouldn't lose hope. And she wanted to stay open-minded to understand and explore all her options, and then make decisions and take action with confidence.

We worked through a few different assessments that I chose specifically based on what she was bringing to the table. With this information we could have a shared understanding of her current identity, personality, and framework. I also gathered information about what actions she had taken with any healthcare providers and what programs of treatment she was currently engaged with. We explored the dynamics of her most prevalent relationships and shed light on old thought-emotion-reaction patterns that were no longer serving her.

Throughout our work together, we did occasional evaluations to give us a measurable sense of incremental progress toward an easing of her struggle and compared these evaluations with her description of how she felt the experience of her journey was changing. The evaluations were in five specific areas of her life that were significant in providing Cathy either support or discouragement.

Our sessions consisted of in-depth discussions of her emotional experiences, practical management of life elements, development of herself within significant relationships, options presented by healthcare providers, identification of further questions that needed answers from healthcare providers, and strategies for staying in the mental-emotional-spiritual space of infinite possibility. I taught Cathy practices for managing her mindset and her physical state. I gave her assignments so she could practice self-care and self-enquiry with the goal that she would eventually not need my coaching.

We addressed Cathy's nutritional practices and how they, in combination with past significant emotional events, were impacting her body and psyche. We designed practices that fit into her life so that she could easily choose what was best for her – what supported and served her in moving toward her visions of what she was becoming and wanted to be experiencing in this life.

The quality of Cathy's life improved overall. And beautifully, after failed IUIs, IVFs and miscarriages, she found her way into being the woman who could hold the possibility of her heart's desire courageously and confidently. She gained the skills to make meaning of significant emotional events in a way that carries her forward instead of holding her back. Now she uses her capacity to generate peace and happiness from the inside out so that she lives more in ease than in struggle. She knows how and she practices daily.

The icing on the cake of Cathy's story is that after all the struggle, the hard clearing work, and then the embodiment of new patterns, she was able to conceive naturally and deliver a healthy baby boy. The elation I feel when a client fulfills her vision, especially one that seems doubtful going in, is hard to put into words. I know her heart burst with joy at having successfully become a mother in a way that she had literally been told was impossible. Even though Cathy's outcome was ideal, there are often magic and miracles to witness in every journey to parenthood, regardless of the outcome.

Conclusion

"When all parts of you connect through the womb, then all parts of you can dance and play together."

**– excerpt from *Womb Wisdom*,
by Padma and Anaiya Aon Prakasha**

Every fertility journey is unique, but all of us share at least one thing: we have felt the powerful coercion of our heart's longing for a baby. And as I've said twice before in this book, your heart gives you a desire not to torture you, but to lead you in the direction of fulfilling the promises of your life. This is true even when you do not get to bring home your baby.

As we move through our journey, encountering the unexpected difficulty of fertility challenges will reveal to us things we never before understood about ourselves. How we react or respond – and these are two very different behaviors – will shape how we experience our passage through this uneven terrain. But how do we equip ourselves with the ability to make as smooth a passage as possible?

I have written this book to help smooth the way. The book cannot erase the pain, but it can offer ease. The book cannot make you pregnant, but it can offer strategies to optimize your fertility. The book cannot answer all your questions, but it can offer you the opportunity to re-engage with and listen to your heart's and body's wisdom. The book cannot erase your fears, but it can renew your hope and feed your courage.

It is my hope and intention that as you read this book, you felt an opening and a shift. You may have noticed the tenor of your experience has changed, even if just slightly.

If you could relate to any part of my story or the descriptions of my clients, you have at the very least gained the knowing that you are not alone. We, and numerous courageous women, have come before you on this turbulent passage toward motherhood. We all make it to the other side; some with babies and some without. The key is in finding our way to the other side still able to enjoy life and live wholeheartedly with all of the trials along the way to either outcome.

I'm finding it hard to leave you here, knowing how many unanswered questions you may still have about your own journey. What I can tell you for sure is that your journey can continue in the frame of struggle with a sense of disempowerment, or it can move into a different frame of ease and empowered forward movement. It is possible that the information in these pages can support you in such a shift. If you want more ease, less struggle, and renewed sense of possibility, it's here for you to choose.

Bibliography and Recommended Reading

Women's Bodies, Women's Wisdom: Creating Physical and Emotional Health and Healing, by Dr. Christiane Northrup

The Other Side of Sadness: What the New Science of Bereavement Tells Us About Life After Loss, by George A. Bonanno

Ended Beginnings: Healing Childbearing Losses, by Claudia Panuthos and Catherine Romeo

Broken Open: How Difficult Times Can Help Us Grow, by Elizabeth Lesser

Re-Membering Lives: Conversations with the Dying and the Bereaved, by Lorraine Hedtke and John Winslade

Power vs. Force: The Hidden Determinants for Human Behavior, by David R. Hawkins, M.D.

The Future of the Body: Explorations into the Further Evolution of Human Nature, by Michael Murphy

Psychoenergetic Science: A Second Copernican-Scale Revolution, by William A. Tiller, Ph.D.

Morphic Resonance: The Nature of Formative Causation, by Rupert Sheldrake

The Hormone Cure, by Sara Gottfried, M.D.

The Mind-Body Fertility Connection: The True Path to Conception, by James Schwartz

Mother from Your Center: Tapping Your Body's Natural Energy for Pregnancy, Birth, and Parenting, by Tami Lynn Kent

The Whole Person Fertility Program: A Revolutionary Mind-Body Process to Help You Conceive, by Niravi B. Payne, M.S. and Brenda Land Richardson

Women's Moods: What Every Woman Must Know About Hormones, The Brain, and Emotional Health, by Deborah Sichel, M.D. and Jeanne Watson Driscoll, M.S., R.N., C.S.

Full Body Living: Love Your Body by Loving Yourself, by Robin Olsen Mayberry

Born to Receive: 7 Powerful Steps Women Can Take Today to Reclaim Their Half of the Universe, by Amanda Owen

Inconceivable: A Woman's Triumph over Despair and Statistics, by Julia Indichova

Taking Charge of Your Fertility: The Definitive Guide to Natural Birth Control, Pregnancy Achievement, and Reproductive Health, by Toni Weschler

The Infertility Cure: The Ancient Chinese Wellness Program for Getting Pregnant and Having Healthy Babies, by Randine Lewis

Acknowledgements

This book has been percolating inside me for a very long time, and birthing it has come in fits and starts like false labor. I am eternally grateful for the encouragement to write that I've had along the way from people who may not have even realized they fed my fire.

The journey to parenthood itself, although painful and soul-shattering at times, is ultimately my blessing. Through all the curious twists of the path, it is only on reflection that I can fully appreciate what I have received in these experiences.

I have deep gratitude for all the women who have shared their stories and their hearts with me in casual conversation and formal survey interviews. And thank you to all the powerful, courageous women I have had the honor and privilege to coach and mentor. You have broadened my understanding of the variety of nuances we experience in the pursuit of parenthood. Through our interactions, we've brought more light to the fact that the only version of normal for the journey to parenthood is the unique experience that each of us has.

The devastation I experienced during the loss of Ava cracked me wide open, and I thank those who helped hold me together while I fell apart, especially those who listened while I repeated the story of my pregnancy, loss, labor, and delivery. Without your compassion and love, I could not have learned to regain compassion and acceptance of myself.

Thank you especially to my beloved life partner and best friend, Scott Pierce. Seeing myself through your eyes was a profound source of courage and strength that carried me through my darkest moments and is still a powerful resource for me today. I am eternally grateful for your stamina, commitment to us, and dedication to what we create together.

I have a special gratitude and place in my heart for a few individuals who in their own special ways have contributed to bringing this book into being. Thank you, Louise Crooks, for helping me understand what I have to offer. Thank you, Susan Engman, for walking me through the darkness. Maggie McReynolds, you are a dear heart, fellow fertility journey veteran, treasured book journey companion, and skilled editor. I am grateful for your guidance and collaboration. Thank you, Angela Lauria, for the Difference Process and Press. You are a truth-teller, powerful leader, and magical mentor.

To the Morgan James Publishing team: Special thanks to David Hancock, CEO & Founder for believing in me and my message. To my Author Relations Manager, Megan Malone, thanks for making the process seamless and easy. Many more thanks to everyone else, but especially Jim Howard, Bethany Marshall, and Nickcole Watkins.

I am also deeply grateful for the time and energy my own mother poured into supporting me and my responsibilities during the highs and lows of the journey. Mom, when the reality I knew became the reality I could no longer deny, you came immediately on the next available flight from across the world to be by my side. What a relief.

Thank you to the powerful teacher and mother-baby advocate, birth educator, and exceptional doula Sharon Muza. I learned so much from you and gained immense strength from you during and after my pregnancies and deliveries – more than you can ever know.

I have special gratitude to Toni Weschler for her expert review of technical details, her encouragement, and conversation. I am honored by the attention you've given this project.

And thank you to all my cheerleaders who encouraged me with their enthusiasm upon learning that I was writing a book and then helped me set it on its way into the world.

About the Author

Julie Pierce is a fertility and healthy lifestyle coach, mother, and wife. Since 1991, she's been on a mission to cut through the dogma and jargon of the healthcare industry and uncover the foundational principles of self-healing and optimal well-being.

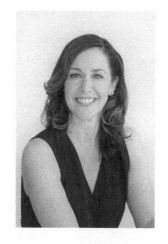

She teaches women how to reclaim their creative power and transform their health from a position of confident choice. When clients work with Julie, both their health and sense of well-being improve. Consequently, everything else in their lives gets better too.

Her own struggles with fertility challenges and other nagging health concerns fueled her dedicated studies in biology, psychology, philosophy, coaching, massage & bodywork, breath work, body intelligence, creative grief work, energy healing, success, feminine power, and mindset research.

Pulling these diverse areas of knowledge and practice together, Julie has designed a methodology that empowers women to identify deepest longings, release binding personal and cultural judgment, and optimize the body and mind's ability to produce desired results.

Julie believes our ability to heal and create is directly related to our ability to receive and cultivate unconditional love. After loss, the experience of unconditional love can become particularly challenging. In relation to fertility, the compounding disappointment of no pregnancy month after month amounts to a deep experience of grief for most women. Her work with those facing fertility challenges, empowers women to return to living wholeheartedly after loss and enables them to release the struggle while continuing to pursue their heart's desire of motherhood with renewed hope and ease. Often, Julie's clients discover that this transformation brings about wholehearted living for the first time since childhood. It's beautiful!

Julie currently resides north of Seattle, Washington. She loves laughing and playing with her 7-year-old son and her life partner of more than 20 years. They share their home and love with a cheeky puppy dog and a persnickety old cat.

Thank You

It is my honor and privilege to share these stories, suggestions, and strategies with you. When a ship shifts its course by as little as one degree, its destination is drastically different, and it's my hope that this book has shifted your course by at least one degree. I am grateful that our paths have intersected.

Throughout this book, I've given you a process of progression that you can follow and implement. The questions that I've posed throughout the text are themselves catalysts in this process. The movement to motherhood, via pregnancy or otherwise, is a movement of shedding an old identity and growing into a new one simultaneously. It can be done in grace or struggle.

Like many journeys, this journey is one of healing. You may have heard the saying, "Healing is a full-time job." You are on that job by choice or otherwise, if that wasn't true you wouldn't be reading this book.

As a thank you present and to offer you support in furthering the ease on your journey while you continue to optimize your fertility, I've created the Fertile Foundations Toolkit which can be found at http://bit.ly/FertTools. In the toolkit you will find:

Quiz: How Fertile Are You?

In this brief quiz mentioned in Chapter 3 – Myths and Miracles of Biochemistry, I walk you through some questions to gauge where you are on the fertility spectrum from a physical perspective. In the results, I give you an overview of how things are right now and some suggestions about what to be considering next.

The Dancing Heart Guided Meditation

In this recorded meditation mentioned in Chapter 11 – Steps: Elements of Shift, I guide you in an exercise of reconnection with your inner wisdom. It's a resource to use as a practice over and over again. You might think of it as a refuge as you cross the stormy sea.

An Opportunity to Connect Directly with Me

As I offered in Chapter 13 – From the Trenches, if you'd like to explore what it could be like to move through your journey to parenthood with more peace in your heart and ease in your life, please join me in a complimentary clarity session. During your session, I will help you get crystal clear about how you can stop struggling and move forward from a place of confident choice again. Most people begin to feel better during the first 15 minutes.

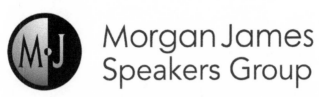

Morgan James
Speakers Group

↗ www.TheMorganJamesSpeakersGroup.com

We connect Morgan James published
authors with live and online events
and audiences who will benefit
from their expertise.

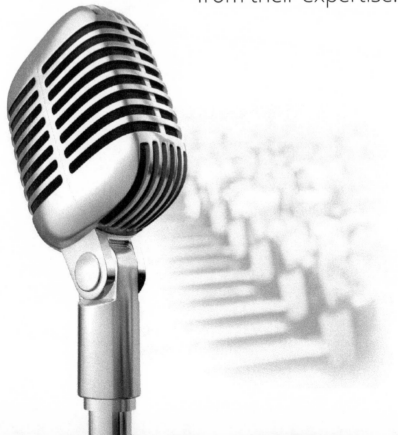